the BIPOLAR DOCTOR

R.T. Kumar, MSc, MD

◆ FriesenPress

Suite 300 - 990 Fort St
Victoria, BC, Canada, V8V 3K2
www.friesenpress.com

Copyright © 2015 by R.T. Kumar

First Edition — 2015

All rights reserved.

No part of this publication may be reproduced in any form, or by any means, electronic or mechanical, including photocopying, recording, or any information browsing, storage, or retrieval system, without permission in writing from FriesenPress.

ISBN
978-1-4602-6574-1 (Hardcover)
978-1-4602-6575-8 (Paperback)
978-1-4602-6576-5 (eBook)

1. Medical, Mental Health

Distributed to the trade by The Ingram Book Company

Contents

v / .... Dedication
vii / .... Introduction
1 / .... Chapter 1
13 / .... Chapter 2
89 / .... Chapter 3
100 / .... Chapter 4
115 / .... Chapter 5
118 / .... Chapter 6
122 / .... Endnotes
124 / .... Appendix 1
126 / .... Appendix 2
128 / .... Appendix 3
131 / .... Appendix 4
132 / .... Appendix 5
135 / .... Appendix 6
137 / .... Sources

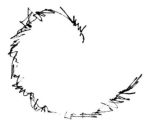

Dedication

I dedicate this book to my mother Janak, who not only taught me the meaning of *true* love but exhibited courage, caring and immense intelligence throughout her life, despite her mental health diagnosis. It is also dedicated to my father who stood by Mom whatever the circumstance, and despite his stubbornness, is the wisest man in the world.

—

Ever since my teens I admired Robin Williams not only for his unique comedic style, but for the realization that he was a true genius in all the academic and lay senses of the word. But as I followed his illustrious career as a physician, personally dealing with mental health disease, and being a physician treating patients with the same ailment, I came to the sad conclusion that this *once in a lifetime individual* was crying out desperately for help, but despite his tremendous means and resources, he received no answers.

I have spent my personal and professional life being recognized as somewhat of a humorous guy, but when on August 11, 2014 I heard that Robin had committed suicide, a significant flame within me was extinguished. My prayers are that the following words may prevent even *one* such tragic event, even more so in an *"everyday"* person, as Robin would have liked it in his *everyman* way and universally agreed upon, unselfish and giving manner.

R.T. Kumar
August 12, 2014

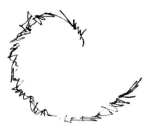

Introduction

Mental health illness – with its prevalence in our society today – affects us all in one way or the other, whether we realize it or not. As the title suggests, the difference is that in this book I describe an experience on how mental health disease affected a doctor and his family, not that we are different from millions of other families.

It wasn't until I became a physician that I truly grasped the stigma, unfairness and neglect directed towards people with a mental health illness. This was not only from my own experience as a doctor with bipolar disorder and depression, but the thousands of mental health patients who have given me the privilege of taking care of them for over twenty-five years.

Some 6.7 million Canadians are living with mental health illness versus 2.2 million with diabetes. Later on in the book I will explain the human, societal and financial cost of this mind-numbing statistic.

—Mental Health Commission of Canada, Making the Case for Investing in Mental Health

My hope is that after reading this book people with mental health problems who have not sought help, or family members who recognize loved ones with symptoms of the disease, will seek medical attention. The consequences of not doing so can sometimes be devastating and cause much unneeded suffering.

In addition, one of the major reasons for me writing this book is to give hope to the millions of people living with mental health diagnoses, revealing the societal hurdles that we have yet to overcome, and hopefully raising awareness among health care professionals, government and the general public about this "endemic" disease. This requires enlightenment, reversal of ignorance, compassion and finally acceptance.

If you take nothing else home from this book, please remember the message about hope at its conclusion in Chapter 6. Hope is inextricably associated with faith (not *necessarily* religion), support from without, determination when it seems you cannot bear another setback (you will!) and most importantly, someone to love and be loved.

As Mother Teresa so aptly put it regarding hope,
"To keep a lamp burning, we have to keep putting oil in it."

the BIPOLAR DOCTOR

R.T. Kumar, MSc, MD

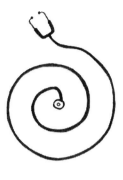

Chapter 1

MY MOTHER

By any measure, my childhood was a very happy one with two very loving parents. We were not affluent but then not lacking for any of the material necessities. My dad was a high school teacher for many years and later a professor at the Canadian Coast Guard College. Mom was intermittently an RN spending most of her working years (after we kids were older) as the head nurse for a multiply-challenged residential facility with violent and troubled patients unable to be kept at home.

We laughed a lot as a family, went on drives almost every day, went to church every Sunday and did yearly short vacations. There was always a "lively" debate going on with our parents who always exhibited an honest interest in our academic and personal lives; sometimes too much so. Mom was the doting mother, always hugging and kissing us even well into our teens.

However, it was at about the age of seven that I began to notice that my mom's behaviour was sometimes very different from other kids' moms. I am four years older than my brother and seven years my sister's senior. When my mother was seven to eight months pregnant with my sister, I recall her staying in bed all day, not cooking for us or doing housework. She wouldn't talk to my brother and me and only seldom with our dad.

HER LIFELONG STRUGGLE WITH DEPRESSION

One day in February when it was so cold that school was postponed (we lived in eastern Canada on the Atlantic Ocean) I vividly remember Mom being very agitated. As our father was a high school teacher at the time, he also had the day off. He told me that he had to go to the doctor urgently that morning and that I should watch my little brother and especially my mom because he was afraid she might try to leave the house. I was a smallish seven-year-old with my mom well over sixty kilograms, being well on in her pregnancy. Sure enough, five minutes after Dad left, Mom tried to force past me and go out into the frigid sub-zero Celsius weather only in her nightie. I was able to hold her off for what seemed like hours, but was only three to four minutes in adult hindsight. Suddenly, she bit me on my stomach. Stunned and having suffered a significant bite, I started to cry, which did nothing but upset my three-year-old baby brother.

Most of this information has been told to me by my father, as I may have not been aware of some of the details and forgotten some facts, due to my age and the trauma of recalling such events. I remember that an officer from the local detachment of the Royal Canadian Mounted Police came to the house when Dad came home, and shortly afterwards a search was started for my mother. She was found forty-five minutes later in a snowdrift and hypothermic.

She was moved to a local hospital where she was stabilized and then moved to a psychiatric hospital eighty kilometres away. When she went into labour about two months later, she was moved to a medical hospital for delivery of my sister and then returned to her psychiatric bed. My aunt took care of my brother, baby sister and me for three months until my mother recovered. My brother and I would sleep at home with my dad at night and spend days after school with our cousins, aunt and uncle.

A common thread throughout my mother's history of depression was that electric shock therapy (ECT or electroconvulsive therapy) usually brought her out of severe depression as per the episode described above. In fact, my mother continued to need ECT until shortly before her death at the age of seventy-two.

This was a particularly severe episode of my mom's lifelong struggle with depression, which is often worsened by pregnancy even in women with no history of psychiatric disease. Post-partum blues, depression and psychosis are a group of conditions that occur in degrees of increasing severity from the former to the latter. The diagnosis of these conditions is still often missed today, and can result in disastrous consequences such as mothers committing suicide and often taking their newborn and other children with them. Although this is thankfully rare, post-partum blues and depression can much more often take a toll on the mother's quality of life and bonding with her newborn and place large amounts of stress on the partner of the affected mother.

Prompt diagnosis of these conditions can lead to very effective treatment and sometimes prevent horrible consequences. In the most severe cases, mothers even require short hospitalizations with their babies as a first stage of recovery from acute psychosis.

In my mom's case, she would stay stable for several years at a time with only medication needed to keep her symptom free. Another crisis arose however when her father died suddenly in a motor vehicle accident in India, with her youngest brother badly injured. In the 1970s, flights could not be arranged as quickly as today, and cremations would occur before North American relatives could reach India. As well, the cost of a flight was prohibitive on my dad's salary as a high school teacher.

In the weeks afterwards, my mother became increasingly withdrawn. Luckily we kids were a lot older – I fourteen years old, my brother ten and my sister two – compared to the episode my mother had at the time of my sister's birth. Unfortunately, she became increasingly despondent and one day, fortunately when we were home, set fire to her mattress in an effort to kill herself. We managed to get the fire out, but Mom was again admitted to hospital for an extended period of time, eventually needing ECT.

Another depression followed the death of her mother, but on this occasion she was able to travel to India, which softened the severity of her disease and did not even need ECT.

I don't want to give the impression that all episodes of depression in people are precipitated by life crises, although we know that stress, lack of sleep and changes in life/work scheduling also contribute. Clinical experience has shown that more often than not, most onsets of depression have no major life event associated with them.[1]

HIGH FUNCTIONING NURSE AND MOTHER

In between these episodes, Mom was a high functioning person, at one period of our lives working full-time shift work at the aforementioned facility as a head nurse, being a full-time mother (a full-time job in itself!) and doing a correspondence degree in health administration. In those days she used a manual typewriter to submit twice monthly lengthy assignments by mail. She did this for over four years. To this day I value this paper degree more than any of the multiple degrees or accolades that I have earned over my career, due to the circumstances under which she earned the degree.

In fact, my mother was the youngest ever Matron (head nurse) of Midwifery at the All India Medical Institutes in New Delhi, the best hospital in India at the time and still one of the most prestigious, where all government officials and the extremely wealthy attend. She also skipped two grades in school; I only one. My point is that a scientific correlation has been made between depression/bipolar disorder and intelligence, creativity and achievement. Probably the best known work on this topic is called *The Creating Brain: The Neuroscience of Genius* by Dr. Nancy Andreasen, a world-renowned psychiatrist and neuroscientist, who prior to this education had a PhD in English literature! She has also been on presidential advisory councils on mental health in the United States as well as too many other distinctions to mention.[2]

Appendix 1 points out several contemporary and historical figures who amply illustrate this scientific correlation. It's as if one gift is given, but something very valuable is taken away in one fell swoop. Tragically, in even these "geniuses in their fields", untreated mental health diagnoses cause greatly diminished quality of life and sometimes more tragic endings. The list of these societal heroes committing suicide increases almost month to month. But what about the *millions* who suffer in silence and anonymity? Hopefully by reading this book some of you in the latter group will, like me, seek help.

A BIT OF FAMILY HISTORY

Over the years we learned some important family history regarding both my mother and my maternal grandmother. My father told me that when he was courting my mother, her mom seemed to be depressed for months at a time. Of course at that time in India – late 1950s early 1960s – depression was not acknowledged let alone treated. It was thought to be God's will or a frailty in one's character. My grandmother's condition deteriorated further when my parents moved to Ethiopia after getting married. It was there that I was born. Eventually, even though we moved to Canada when I was two years old, my grandmother improved with time. What her ongoing life history with depression was, was never discussed.

This seemingly "spontaneous" resolution of my grandmother's and the majority of cases of mild depression can be explained. Most cases of mild depression get better with time as the neurotransmitters that are lacking in the disease get replenished by the brain without intervention. However, without treatment, these depressive episodes become more frequent, last longer and are more resistant to spontaneous recovery as the neurotransmitter-making cells "get tired". Starting the correct anti-depressant medication can decrease the frequency of episodes, decrease the time to recovery and generally improve the quality of life.

CRISIS-INDUCED RECOVERY?

I was in second year university and my mother was in a psychiatric hospital for another exacerbation of her depression, when my father had a heart attack at the age of forty-six. My fourteen-year-old brother and eleven-year-old sister were living with family friends with both of my parents hospitalized. I came home from university a week or two before Christmas exams to do the little I could.

What was amazing is that normally Mom's recovery, even with ECT, would have taken weeks to months. However, with her husband in a condition where he needed her urgently, she made a miraculous recovery within days, and was at home taking care of *all* of his needs, as well as doing things that would have normally been his purview, for example paying bills, doing home repairs, doing heavy work around the house, etc.

It is amazing how some depressed patients make rapid recoveries when life circumstances dictate. Although no studies have been done, I would conjecture that an override switch must cause rapid production of neurotransmitters somewhat similar to a "fight or flight" response. Maybe if we understood this phenomenon better, improved anti-depressant treatments could be designed.

On the whole, Mom remained healthy as I moved to Germany for graduate studies and then returned to Canada for medical school. My mother had the same psychiatrist for over thirty years.

This has its advantages and downfalls. On one hand, the doctor gets to know his patient very well, with their history, response to treatments and so on. On the other hand, long time psychiatrists may become complacent, not keep in touch with the latest treatment modalities as they age, and "lose the forest for the trees" in new symptom presentations and nuances in the mental health status that require attention.

One example was when my mother was visiting my wife and I after I had been practicing medicine for about five years. I had not seen her for one year. I noticed immediately that her gait was different *(petit pas–* small steps in French), her movements rigid and obvious tremors. It would have been obvious to a first year medical student that she was exhibiting classic symptoms of Parkinson's disease. Unfortunately, none of her doctors had noticed the symptoms as they all had been her doctors for such a long time (family doctor and psychiatrist). I immediately told my parents about the medications that she needed and that the symptoms were due to her psychiatric medications. At that time, depression medications could have been used that would have avoided the Parkinsonian symptoms. In the end, the decision was made by her psychiatrist to continue her present depression medications but add Parkinson's medications on top of things. The combination of these drugs of course had a new set of side effects, but she tolerated them.

Around this time, my mother's youngest brother from California visited my parents in Nova Scotia from where he had emigrated from India. I was only able to come home for a couple of days due to practice obligations, but since we were both ex-military, we formed a quick bond. (He had not seen me since I was an infant.)

He told me about the closeness he had shared with my mother as kids. My paternal grandfather was quite the disciplinarian and my uncle had formed a friendship with the son of one of the servants. Such a liaison would have been impossible had my grandfather known. My mom was so close with him that she would make excuses for my uncle when he was playing with his friend. One night my uncle was just sneaking back into the house from a rendezvous with his chum when he was caught by my grandfather. My mom was so protective of my uncle that she took the blame for the whole affair, including the thrashing that accompanied it.

With these stories my uncle also related a more serious event in my mother's history.

THE DARK UNDERBELLY OF THE PARTITION OF INDIA

Partition was a horrible event in India and Pakistan's history, where people who had lived in harmony for hundreds of years became enemies almost overnight, on the grounds of religion and fanatical nationalism. Literally millions of people passed each other going in opposite directions of dirt lanes separated by grass medians with all of the belongings that they could carry on their backs. They were headed for the *correct* nation based solely on their religious affiliation. Occasionally, savage violence would break out with either Hindu or Muslim instigators exposing onlookers to savagery beyond description.

My uncle retold of how his family had to leave Lahore, that was about to become Muslim Pakistan, and move to India, the new state for Hindus. My maternal grandfather was a wealthy businessman who had to abandon all that he had worked so hard for during his lifetime and leave Lahore in a hurry to save his family's lives.

About two hours after the family of five children, my grandparents and several servants and their families fled from their home, it was realized that a crucial immigration document was forgotten. It was decided that my teenage mother, although the middle child, was the most trustworthy to go back with a servant to pick up the documents. Apparently their return was quite delayed. According to her younger brother (the uncle relating the story to me) and independently from my mother's older sister, my mother's happy-go-lucky demeanour was never the same after this episode. It was not much longer after that she started to develop depressive episodes.

It was known that widespread rape and physical assault was perpetrated by both sides in the process of partition. It is my and my mother's siblings conjecture that something happened on that trip back to retrieve documents. Whether it was a sexual assault, emotional abuse, etc., no one is sure. The likelihood of anyone approaching my mother in those days or asking what happened are remote. No one has tried to ask her since.

We know that although some mental health problems have a large genetic component, traumatic life events can certainly make a major contribution. The percentage contribution of each of the above are a debate found in many aspects of human disease, that is nature vs. nurture. For example, it is well established that over 90 per cent of eating disorders (anorexia nervosa/bulimia nervosa) are related to a sexual abuse history in those patients, whether they be male or female. Unfortunately these illnesses remain amongst the hardest to treat in psychiatry and need lifelong care and courageous perseverance for patients with the diagnosis.

Therefore the part that early life trauma played in my mother's mental state remains unknown to this day.

The course of my mother's depression was fairly stable after my dad's heart attack. She was always complaining to us kids about dad's non-compliance with his diet and diabetes, as if a word from any of us, even "the doctor" in the family, would have made any difference! Outside the slowing that comes with normal aging, Mom seemed to be doing okay. I must admit that I became a bit over engaged in my life and career and may not have noticed changes in her psychiatric health. I think it also sort of crept up on my dad who himself was in his seventies, and my brother who now lived at home with my parents. At any rate, I one day received a call from my dad saying that Mom had been admitted to hospital with severe depression. We communicated on a weekly basis and I remember thinking that this seemed to have come out of nowhere.

A SAD CASE OF CHRONIC MEDICAL NEGLECT

Mom apparently stopped eating on the psychiatric ward and no one informed the family. Despite my father and brother's efforts to feed her, she had very little intake. Intravenous lines were not allowed on the "psych" floor and she eventually also became dehydrated. I do not have the patient records, but I am quite certain that Mom's kidney function would have started to suffer.

What happens to patients' stomachs when they get no food for prolonged periods of time is that the lining thins until a blood vessel is exposed and bleeds. That is why patients in the Intensive Care Unit (ICU) on a ventilator are always on medications to decrease stomach acid production and have food through tubes in their nose or by intravenous with prolonged dependence on a machine to help them breathe (vent for short).

Apparently this no-food situation went on for a long time with Mom until disastrous consequences occurred.

My mother went on to have a massive stomach bleed, and while in the operating room went into cardiac arrest. We have never as a family have been able to find out how often she was shocked to restart her heart, or "how long she was down" with no blood flow to her brain. Before the event she was speaking very little to my dad and brother, but after the arrest she never spoke again.

She was transferred to a "medical floor" where my father and brother discovered that the nurses/nurses aids would spend less than two or three minutes trying to feed Mom and then give up and leave. She was left for extended times in her own feces and urine and eventually developed bed sores. I wish that I could say my mother's situation is isolated, but over the years have heard hundreds of families of my patients say exactly the same thing. The reasons for such travesties of human dignity are complicated, having to do with staff shortages, apathy of staff resulting from patient abuse and hospital politics and infighting. Regardless of the cause, their occurrence is inexcusable.

My father was incensed, especially since neglect had landed his wife in this tragic mess. Fortunately, he was good friends with the medical director of the hospital who we had known socially for thirty years. I had also gone to school with his son for years and the director knew that I was a physician now. I had in fact worked the emergency room under this director for one year.

Despite all this, the situation perhaps even worsened. I often wonder how she would have been treated if we didn't "have all the ins". In other words, how do *ordinary people* with no connections and means learn about what is really going on with their loved ones with psychiatric disease. In addition, there were at least fifteen to twenty physicians in the city, both specialists and family doctors, who had personally known our family for thirty to thirty-five years and peeked in on her and checked in with my dad from time to time.

My father hired a private personal care worker to feed Mom while she was in hospital. However he found that even this was ineffective, and in his early seventies he came once daily to feed her while my brother did another meal. All this was done with a ten to fifteen kilometre drive through rain and snow every day, season by season, and my father risking his own fragile health in a cesspool of germs daily. (In fact, a nationally-recognized independent survey indicated that this very hospital had a higher than average death rate of surgical patients post-operatively by infection!) They stayed by her bedside for hours while she didn't talk. Finally a feeding tube had to be put in her nose and eventually after that kept on being pulled out, a feeding tube was put directly into her stomach through the skin (gastrostomy tube).

As is then typical for mental health patients, the bed that was being occupied by my mother was needed for a real "medical patient", although she could not have been more of a medical patient! The real reason, admitted by the administration, was that she was really a "psychiatric" patient occupying a medical bed. This happens in hospitals daily, nationally and in the U.S., due to a myriad of health care issues: fiscal cuts, bed management shortfalls and physicians not moving patients *out* of hospital in efficacious manners. The topic itself is enough for an entire book!

My father was naturally furious and in his frustration over substandard care in the hospital, decided to take Mom home. This was no small feat, as he had to purchase a hospital bed (luckily partly covered by medical insurance), hire private nurses up and beyond the once daily short nursing visit allowed by government insurance, feed my mother three times daily since the gastrostomy tube had to be taken out (a task shared by my brother who lived at home) and change diapers as needed. This was again daunting and commendable in his love for Mom, reiterating once more, he was a man in his seventies with active heart disease, kidney disease and diabetes. My brother however was a Godsend in the help he gave the two of them in this regard.

The two of them persisted on with Mom for over one and a half years, showing their unending dedication to her mental health needs and overwhelming medical diagnoses. This type of dedication is seen in many families who at times have been "abandoned" by the medical establishment and have to make do in tragic situations. Luckily "we" had some knowledge of medicine and were strong advocates for my mom.

One morning, my brother was feeding her breakfast and she swallowed wrong and started to cough violently. An ambulance was called immediately, but she died despite resuscitation efforts before she reached the hospital. It was not a comfortable way to die, how much I appreciate, you will read on. But it was relatively quick and beat the much diminished quality of life she had been experiencing for almost three years.

Our mental health care system failed my mother and our family in many ways.

Such tragedies are not sadly unknown. Thousands of patients and families like ours are let down in this same way each year.

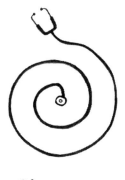

Chapter 2

THE BIPOLAR DOCTOR – ME

As previously mentioned, I was blessed with a very happy childhood having been born in Ethiopia and immigrated to Canada in 1965.

I was precocious and inquisitive and in Grade 1, the guidance counsellor at my elementary school called in my parents for a chat. Basically they said I was totally unchallenged in my present grade and therefore could be disruptive with my talking (a habit I have to this day, ha, ha!). I had undergone IQ testing (for what that's worth) unbeknownst to me and my parents, and it indicated that I was in a "genius" range especially in linguistic, reading and mathematics ability. They wanted me to skip from first to third grade. A lot of discussion went on between my parents, administration and teachers about my ability to handle the social change, my level of maturity and adaptive capacity. My mother had skipped two grades as I have mentioned and my parents thought that I could handle the change.

I was like a fish taking to water, made many friends and was challenged to a slightly greater degree academically. Things went on swimmingly. Unfortunately I was also a victim of what I like to call the "East Indian My Kid Should be a Doctor Syndrome"!

It may be disrespectful, but I often say in a tongue in cheek manner that many Indian parents would rather have a doctor as a child than a Prime Minister! There is certainly some hyperbole in this statement, but the sentiment is clear I think, and would be verified by a lot of first generation Indo-Canadian kids.

Well my story was a bit more complicated. When we first came to Canada in 1965, there was a famous aspirin commercial with a 'doctor' who said, "Take two aspirin and call me in the morning." Well don't ask me if it was subliminal suggestion by my parents or my own free will, but from the age of three I wanted to become a doctor! In all seriousness! At the age of two to three I could recite the scheduling of any television program for my dad (my TV watching buddy) on the only two stations available then, for the entire week 5:00 p.m. to 11:00 p.m. That thinking capability in part, *may* have shown that I had enough understanding about the seriousness of my desire for my future career! Or maybe not.

Others may argue that was just a rote memory skill, but I beg to differ as this strong desire persisted to the day I said the Hippocratic Oath!

However, as much as my parents denied it, there was always a huge pressure to be the best academically. As reverse racist or realistic as it was, it was drilled into my head that because we were immigrants, I had to be twice as good as a Canadian-born, Caucasian student. That thought stayed with me lifelong and had a definite negative impact on my development as an adult and even at times precipitated depression periodically through my life I think.

The pressure definitely became a self-imposed one as the years went by, but caused me to want to achieve more, which led to fatigue, which brought on depression, which worsened the depression because I was not achieving. A scary cycle. My *curriculum vitae* and LinkedIn profile, a website for all sorts of professionals worldwide Appendix 4, reveals this never-ending desire to achieve was associated with little fulfillment or happiness as you will see.

A BRIEF DIGRESSION ...

Unfortunately, many mental health patients never achieve their desires in life because their depression is never treated or even recognized. However, as has already been mentioned in the context of Dr. Andreasen, and Appendix 1 *only a few* of the famous people who have struggled with their mental health were recognized as having an illness, yet achieved so much in all spheres of human achievement. That is to say, how many of the approximately twenty to twenty-five per cent of the general population with a mental health diagnosis are "geniuses in waiting", not recognized as such because of the stigma of mental health in our society, its lack of diagnosis and treatment?

My biggest frustration is how many Winston Churchills, Michelangelos, Sir Isaac Newtons, Van Goghs, Beethovens, Abraham Lincolns, Isaac Newtons, Charles Dickens, Ernest Hemingways, Jim Carreys, Billy Joels, Harrison Fords, Buzz Aldrins and Robin Williams (see acknowledgements) to only name a handful, are out there.

Even these people admired by society and history had disease greatly affecting their lives, which remained undiscovered under their façades of greatness. Beneath are several pathetic layers of sadness, hopelessness, utter futility and sometimes tragedy, despite the abundance of resources available to them (not prior to the early twentieth century), and perhaps the ignorance of onlookers around them. This latter statement *has* to be qualified, as sometimes symptoms are hidden by the patient, atypical or not recognizable to the lay person or even health professional. *But*, not bringing a loved one to medical attention, sometimes very much against their will when the symptoms are blatant and prolonged, is ignorance in my very biased opinion. As is pointed out repeatedly, the consequences of inaction are often irreversible and grievous. Of course even when help is sought, the medical *system* often fails.

BACK TO THE STORY

Things were progressing well despite the pressure I felt to achieve when suddenly at the age of fifteen I began to require less sleep, seemed to have great amounts of mental energy, became more irritable and generally was not myself. I spoke back at school to the vice principal and only by my father's diplomatic skills was not suspended. This from a kid with a straight 'A' average since Grade 1 until now in Grade 11, and never admonished for any misbehaviour.

I suddenly spent the majority of my savings on an electric guitar amp when I only had an acoustic guitar. I became more sexual towards girls (not overtly but relatively) at school where I was normally the shyest of nerds (even compared to Sheldon on The Big Bang Theory!). I became *more* talkative than normal, the subjects and flow of my speech not that coherent. Usually I prided myself on my glib and erudite manner. However most distressing to my parents, was that I was not listening to them at all, which I mostly did, usually more than the average teenage boy.

MY FIRST MEDICAL 'INCARCERATION'

My parents became very concerned especially with my mother's psychiatric history, and discussed it with our family physician and mother's psychiatrist. The decision was made to bring me to the outpatient department of our local hospital under some other context, sedate me and send me to the provincial psychiatric hospital three hundred kilometres away by ambulance and in restraints. I don't remember much about the trip (I was pretty loopy!) but when I arrived at the hospital I remember everyone being very cold. One sentence questions. No concern expressed, and then I was left alone in an empty room for what seemed like hours. When he came in, the doctor was in his late fifties or early sixties I would imagine, and was in a white lab coat (I suppose appropriate enough when as a lay person you always heard of white straight-jackets in such places!) and spoke in a very matter of fact manner. To my non-doctor ear he was asking a lot of questions unrelated to my life at the time.

I guess we spoke for about fifteen to twenty minutes then a male attendant took me to a locked ward and a room with two felony criminals awaiting psychiatric observation to gauge fitness to stand trial. I was "thrilled" being this innocent kid from smalltown eastern Canada. One was a typical biker (forgive the stereotype) who was charged with attempted murder. He was about five foot ten inches and must have weighed over two hundred fifty pounds and covered with tattoos like a book cover. He said very little except at medication times where he complained about everything he was on, which was obviously a chemical restraint. Within a few days he learned his medications (meds) were giving him quite the buzz, so in exchange for extra dessert I would "cheek" my meds and give them to him. He became more buzzed, I felt safer and had extra dessert two meals a day.

The other patient was diametrically opposite to patient one. He was tall and lanky with lesser but an impressive array of tattoos. I can't remember what he was "in for" (sounds like prison, which it was) but he talked incessantly. The two reminded me of that Bugs Bunny cartoon where a big tough bulldog ambled down the street with this yappy small dog, who is constantly irritating the larger canine with useless banter, and gets an abrupt backhand from time to time from the big dog with an accompanying "Ahh *shut up*" in a Brooklyn accent. In the end, when the big dog was challenged by some wild big cat and the little dog went in behind the same gate with a kitten there now, instead of the wild, ferocious cat, the relationship switched with the big bulldog being the hanger-on and the small dog the alpha canine! Classic Mel Blanc!

There was never any switching of roles with these two and they turned out to be quite nice guys for felons.

I soon found out that I was the youngest patient there on the ward with the next person at least ten years older (years later special adolescent wards would be built). I benefited from a certain bit of kid glove treatment, which quickly ended when the staff noted no change in my hypomanic condition despite medication. The diversion trick was discovered and from then on I had witnessed liquid doses of medications.

The definition of hypomania versus mania is difficult even in medical jargon. Suffice it to say my cover was blown and my big felon buddy wasn't as buzzed as he wanted to be, luckily not to the detriment of my physical health.

I hated my father for weeks for bringing me to this horrible place against my will. The first signs of my recovery were as this "teenage hate" dissipated. In hindsight, as a physician who has treated his share of mental health patients, I was put on a medication called Perphenazine, which belongs to a class known as typical antipsychotics. This drug had several nasty side effects such as movements of the body and face with no control, lockjaw and moderate to severe clouding of the mind making ordinary school thinking difficult. I ended up in the ER on several occasions with severe trismus (unable to open jaw) requiring a shot. Of course the Cogentin, the drug against trismus, made you quite drowsy, which wasn't helpful for an adolescent in high school trying to navigate the perils of puberty and at the same time excel in school to "become a doctor". (Cogentin was given all the time with the Perphenazine in tablet form and additional doses by shot when the lockjaw occurred in the emergency room setting.)

BACK TO SCHOOL

After several weeks in hospital I returned to school. I'm unsure now about what excuse I gave about my tumultuous return. Kids being kids though they forgot about why "the brain" had been gone, my myriad of extra-curricular activities continued, though my school grades were significantly lower that year.

My mental health follow-up was horrible. It consisted of five-minute "chats" with my mother's psychiatrist of twenty years, who knew little about my diagnosis as he never changed my treatment in the face of my mother's well-established history. That is, he never changed me to chronic bipolar or even depression treatment. I never did see the doctor who put me on the drugs in the hospital in the first place.

Gradually over a year the drugs were discontinued.

I graduated from high school with one of the highest averages ever seen in December when decisions were made for scholarships. I received a good amount of money on the basis of my marks and was accepted to a respectable undergraduate program in science that had a medical school. In the second half of my final year of high school I had no interest in studying and did not crack a book, likely with some rebound depression, having been not treated for same. At any rate I finished with an average of ninety and made the Honour Roll with *no* studying whatsoever.

The next five years were uneventful from the point of view of my depression. I ate my way through first year university putting on 'the freshman fifteen', except in my case it was thirty pounds. My marks went from straight A's in high school to B's and C's. I was so paranoid about the mark situation and expectations for medical school, that I forged them to send them to my parents who suffered with terminal "my kid needs to get to medical school syndrome!"

In the first half of second year my mother was back in the hospital and my father had a sudden heart attack at the age of forty-six. Luckily it was not too severe, but it left a fourteen-year-old brother and eleven-year-old sister at home alone. I quickly made arrangements with my professors and borrowed money for a flight home. After a few harried days of visiting my dad in the coronary care unit and Mom in the psychiatric hospital, I somehow kept it together for my siblings. Through some wonderful friends, food and child care was arranged for the kids. As I mentioned earlier, my mother made a miraculous recovery within days of the heart attack and took on tasks that she never managed in her lifetime.

I did miserably at Christmas with a D in organic chemistry, ironically a subject my father taught! He later told me that he was happy that I almost failed because after a lifetime at excelling at everything I did, I had to learn about failure at something that was really of no consequence.

Third year of university was much more successful with my average back up to about a B+, A- and A's. It still wasn't enough to get into medical school though. I subsequently decided to do my Honours in Microbiology/Molecular Genetics. A West German (at that time) professor was very impressed with my marks and enthusiasm in third year and invited me to do my Honour's degree with a group of Germans she was bringing to Canada with two post-graduate fellows from the U.K. (who had their PhDs already). Eventually that led to me going to Germany, not only being able to do some cutting-edge research ("cloning" as the fledgling science was called), learning a new language and culture *and* falling in love for the first time.

M. was a very atypical German, playing jokes, teasing, always smiling. It was some time before we started dating in earnest, when I learned that I had been accepted to medical school. It was one of the most heart-wrenching things I ever had to do, leaving the first woman to whom I truly could say "I love you" and have to start one of the most challenging and hard times in my life (so I thought).

MEDICAL SCHOOL AND THE CANADIAN ARMED FORCES

We had the tearful goodbye at the airport and then weekly phone calls with alternating biweekly letters (prior to email, text and twitter) ensuing. The summer after first year medical school I went back to Germany to finish off some research. We reunited, and this fiercely patriotic, strong family person, announced that she wanted to leave her family and join me in Canada. We got married in second year medical school.

It was this same year that I applied and was accepted to the Canadian Armed Forces Medical Officers' Training Plan (MOTP). This plan consisted of the Forces financing second, third and fourth year medical school along with internship with three years of military service as a doctor in return.

Any doctor will tell you that up to that point in their life, medical school was the most difficult experience taking into consideration physical, emotional, academic and relationship stressors. We now know that significant numbers of trainees suffer from mental health disorders that may have been there prior entry to medical school, and may have even ironically helped get them into this close fraternity! However the stress of training may bring the disorders on as well.

I did well until third year when I had finished the most stressful first and second years, and was about to embark on the fun of third year, where we began to have meaningful relationships with patients. At the end of this period we had full year exams covering everything that we had learned over that time frame. As third year came to a close, I found myself becoming more tired, less motivated (poison to a medical student), ambivalent to sex (with a new and beautiful wife), requiring increased sleep, having little interest in activities of enjoyment (sports, exercise, TV, etc.) and an overwhelming feeling to stay in bed all day.

Both my wife and I became concerned and went to a wonderful help program provided by the medical school. I was referred to a great family doctor who was in his retiring years of practice. He diagnosed exhaustion. No diagnosis of depression was made and I was given two to three weeks off to recuperate and took the exams a month later than my colleagues. As I have mentioned earlier, my neurotransmitters in a state of depression likely recharged on their own and the "exhaustion" cured itself.

The rest of third and fourth year went well despite long hours of being on call without sleep, a factor often associated with bringing on depression in people with known disease. I also noted that sometimes when others of my colleagues were shutting down with fatigue at 3:00 a.m., I had tons of energy to go on working. I would feel bursts of energy that were like what kids feel on Christmas morning and it was good!

THE IRRITABLE INTERN

I finished medical school and then went into internship, which was probably the most grueling part of the training, where staying up on call for twenty-four hours every third night was the norm, and sometimes being up for thirty-six hours every second night, when someone was on holiday.

As internship progressed, I found this "high" very useful and didn't really see any side effects. However, my wife and some colleagues noticed that I was becoming irritable from things that were totally out of proportion with regards to the stimulus and the response. I would snap at colleagues, something that I never would have done under normal circumstances. After a thirty-six hour shift my wife would take care of everything in the house (as she did all our life together and all I did was study). If by chance she asked me to take out heavy garbage, for example I often would snap back with a comment like, "Doesn't working twenty-four hours without a break stand for something?" This was very different from the way our relationship really was, where I tried to be as supportive of her with her entire family on the other side of the world.

M. would rightfully be insulted and hurt especially since more often than not *she* had put in a twelve-hour day between her very complicated career in medical research, commuting two hours return from work, and then all the chores at home that she did in my long absences at the hospital. She was really a trooper.

We managed to get by however, until an incident with some visitors we were entertaining from Europe. They were the very good friends of ours with whom we had done research in both Canada and then when I had traveled to Germany for my Master's degree. I had lived with one of them without rent for two years and they both became like older brothers to me when I had arrived in Germany, six or seven years earlier, a young Canadian, first time in a foreign country, foreign language and not so subtle racism towards visible minorities. Bavaria where I lived was at the time the most conservative state in the West Germany. I owed them a lot really.

In an ironic twist of fate, I literally saved one of them as he was actively contemplating suicide one day, leaving my research lab that day on "a hunch" well before I was a doctor. I suppose my experience with Mom gave me some insight. He was a victim of depression in a culture that, at least in the mid-eighties, was considered more a character weakness than illness. I think his sister who was a nurse and worked in psychiatry knew of his condition, but was unable to do anything because of his denial. I did tell her about this gesture and I think she did get him help, as his mood improved tremendously over the next few months.

However with this "new irritability", I made their trip quite miserable. I did take them to Niagara Falls with M. where we had a good time, and toured the sights of Toronto quite successfully. All I remember is one night I had a disagreement with them both over some trivial subject and ended up sleeping in my call room at the hospital, which was only half a kilometre from our house.

The next morning they were re-booking their ticket back to Germany two days early. Despite the fact that all these events were happening while I was actively training in the medical field, it never dawned on me that *my* behaviour was being affected by a mental health diagnosis.

We managed to survive the rest of my internship and I was accepted to do a year of Internal Medicine training sponsored by the military but counting towards one year of my payback service. We moved again back to the city where I went to medical school. Unfortunately the time apart due to me being on call was still significant, and my responsibilities as a doctor specializing in Internal Medicine increased.

My wife's loneliness and missing her family peaked, even though we visited them in Germany every chance we had.

She therefore invited her younger sister, with whom she had had a very close relationship while at home, and the sister's fiancé for a two week visit to Canada. I was going to work for one week while she toured with them locally and then we were going to visit my parents 300 km away and stay at a quaint country resort for a few days and then slowly drive back home seeing the sights.

That was the plan anyway.

I remember having been on call the night before we were to leave, having only got two to three hours of sleep. I slept for a few hours and we then set off for the first 300 km leg of our trip. My wife sat in the back seat of our small hatchback with her sister, engaging in "girl" talk, while us men were in the front seat. I spoke fluent German with the fiancé, which wasn't *the* problem.

However what was a problem was the differing political views in the front seat. For some background, this was the time after the first five years of the Berlin Wall having come down. The affluent West Germans (my in-laws) now had a stream of East Germans flooding across the borderless frontier taking "West" jobs, often for much lower wages. In addition, the "West" Germans now looked at the ever present immigrant populations as a threat. For example, at that time in Munich where I lived, about three per cent of the city's population were Turkish.

The Turks had been brought in during the fifties and sixties to do a lot of the menial labour jobs that local Germans did not want to do in rebuilding the war-ravaged country. There were now two to three generations of Turks in Bavaria (province of which Munich was the capital) who may have been living off social assistance, living two to three families in an apartment and renting the social assistance subsidized housing to lower socio-economic Germans who enjoyed no such social benefits.

The animosity this caused is self-evident. However what may not be so clear, is that Bavaria was a stronghold and arguably the starting point for Adolph Hitler's drive to lunacy. The academic people that I associated with in my research were ashamed of this portion of their history almost to an obsessive-compulsive pitch. However amongst the blue collar Bavarians open racism was not only present but resulted in open Neo-Nazi organization (crushed by the state and federal governments) and even election of ultra-Conservative rightist parties at the state or provincial level in Bavaria. (The fiancé that I was sitting with was decidedly blue collar and an ultra-Conservative!) These were scary facts for a visible minority who was treated as a Turk while living in Germany and worse now, married to a "native" German.

I must add at this point, that at no time in my marriage to M. was race an issue. Her great-uncles some of whom were Nazi soldiers in the war gave me great big bear hugs welcoming me to the family, and we raised more than a few *masse* (one litre mugs of beer you see at Oktoberfest, ten to twelve of which are being carried by a small but mighty barmaid!) together.

One of the greatest lessons I learned from being married to M. was that although a good number of Germans were brainwashed by Hitler's xenophobic ramblings, a very large number had to go along in order to protect the lives of their loved ones who were always being watched by the crazy dictator's minions. I discovered this for myself in my relationships with the dozens of in-laws I met on both the East and West side of Germany.

Now although I sometimes stray off topic there is always a logical explanation! While I sat in the seat next to my sister-in-law's fiancé, we started to discuss the political situation in the unified Germany. Eventually the conversation turned to the presence of immigrants in the country and their effect on German-born citizens. He became very "rabid" in his conversation and I have to admit that I also became agitated with his quasi-racist comments and we got into it.

As it continued on, I think I became hypomanic and drove faster. The more my speed increased the more irate my wife and sister-in-law became. It came to the point that I pulled off the road with both my wife and sister-in-law in tears. We got through the rest of the drive in silence until we reached my parents' house where we were to overnight. My wife and I had an earnest talk about the day, and with my mood altered by the mania, I made the unreasonable decision to not participate in the resort visit, but stay with my parents, play golf and then fly back to where we lived.

HYPOMANIA AND THE END OF MY FIRST MARRIAGE

My wife was devastated but despite her pleas I persisted with my stubborn plan.

The three went on to stay on plan for their visit and returned one morning while I was away starting a thirty-two hour call in the hospital.

The next morning I opened the door to the house and was shocked to see that all my wife's belongings were gone, fifty per cent of the joint savings were withdrawn and she had quit her job. No one at her workplace would divulge her whereabouts to me but I was able to trace the flights back to Germany for my wife, sister-in-law and brother-in-law. However, in the interim I was served with divorce papers citing irreconcilable differences as the basis for separation. I was therefore unable to see her prior to her departure back to Germany.

All this transpired over forty-eight hours. Typical German efficiency at work.

The suddenness with which everything happened stunned me, and even though I was a doctor in his late twenties with a job with considerable responsibility, I just wanted to have my parents by my side. My brother who lived in the same city came over that night to keep me company until my parents arrived the next day.

I vividly remember bursting into tears when my mom came into the house, and laying on the sofa next to her as she stroked my head and I fell into a deep sleep. When I awoke I felt rested but obviously still sad. I remember ironically that one of the things that bothered me the most, was that I had failed in one of life's major tasks; one that I had idyllically always viewed as lifelong, having only ever had my parents' rock solid example through thick and thin.

Also, I had never failed "academically or intellectually" in any of life's challenges. This all came to me as an added blow in addition to the sudden separation, with my wife having moved to the other side of the world, not amenable to any face-to-face reconciliation attempts.

I had a very understanding commanding officer (CO), an exception for the military as I will outline in another chapter, who gave me as much time off as I needed. I returned to work in a few days and my parents returned home.

Over the next seven to ten days I began to drink more alcohol (usual for me was two to three drinks weekly, now I was drinking two to three drinks *per night*). I understandably started to get a lot of heartburn, to the point that my CO, who was an Internal Medicine specialist decided to look inside my stomach and first part of my intestine with a scope. He found some early signs of wear on the lining of my stomach (gastritis) and put me on the strongest stomach protection medications at the time. He also told me to decrease my alcohol intake, which was kind of a joke considering the mentality of alcohol use and the military.

I managed to get to work daily and do my job as an Internal Medical trainee. It was as demanding as internship, with often me being the only doctor in house overnight for the specialty, and over hundreds of patients on service, many quite ill. The stress was great and the ongoing mourning over my failed marriage continued. I even flew to Germany and stayed at a hotel trying to convince my still wife (only three months since separation) to come back. Things were very civil, with her parents being supportive of my cause, but the damage had been done.

I returned to Canada with only having been gone three days including travel.

MENTAL HEALTH DIAGNOSES IN THE CANADIAN MILITARY

I slowly started to have problems sleeping, with fatigue, early morning waking and irritability very unusual for me. I was in a particularly demanding rotation and suddenly one day felt that I couldn't cope. I went to my family doctor and after some consultation it was felt that I had reactionary depression due to my marital separation (first of the several mistakes to be made in my diagnosis over decades!).

At that time in the military, early 1990's, mental health diagnoses were often not made. In fact the advice was to "suck it up" soldier and move on. A stiff belt was also often not discouraged. I was consulted to a very understanding and knowledgeable psychiatrist but had to sneak into appointments so that none of the other hospital personnel, most were subordinates to me in the military ranks, would see me. He started me on a brand new class of drugs called SSRIs. The first drug was one called Zoloft, which he warned might make me irritable. Well it sure did, as I yelled at some subordinate colleagues and a distinct change in behaviour was noted by all. I was almost always very upbeat and the "Hawkeye" of the unit harkening back to the 1970s comedy of army life and being a physician. I often tried to buck military regulations to help my patients and made light of the ludicrous administration.

It must be remembered that it was made clear to every person enlisted in the military you signed off your "human rights" as we know them in civilian life. Therefore your medical record was an open book to any superior. We as physicians were very cognizant of this and would sometimes "not include clinical details" on patients to combat this breech of patient-doctor confidentiality and affect their rank progression, often starting anti-depressant meds.

Well the irritability with Zoloft was another misdiagnosis that would take years to straighten up. I was eventually put on Prozac and this drug worked much better, and within weeks I was back to being my usual positive, irreverent military doctor self!

Unfortunately, after months the drug was discontinued, as continuing on it decreased my functional ability as a soldier, that is I could not be posted to a combat or high stress job on anti-depressants. This was about the time Canada was being asked to participate in more active theatres such as "Desert Storm", Bosnia, Somalia, Haiti and Rwanda. Doctors were especially needed in these missions for obvious reasons.

Thus was yet another mistake in the management of my "depression" that is very commonly made even today.

I continued well through the rest of my military career, even becoming the medical director of the Addiction Rehabilitation Clinic (ARC) Atlantic. This clinic served about 70 per cent of the Canadian Navy, thousands of Army and Air Force personnel east of Quebec, and Canadian Forces Europe and all other theatres worldwide. To say that I was privy to the suffering of thousands of people through substance dependence is an understatement. But the thing that distressed me the most is that it is generally agreed that 90 per cent of substance dependent people have a concomitant mental health disorder (substance dependence already being one), depression, anxiety disorders, bipolar disease and Post Traumatic Stress Disorder (PTSD) being the most common ones.[3]

The sad thing is the prognosis of addiction recovery significantly decreases with the severity of mental health diagnoses, with almost all addicts, in my experience, having had severe psychological, physical or sexual traumas that can often manifest as PTSD later on in life.[4] The majority of our ARC patients did not receive a psychiatric diagnosis let alone treatment for these ailments, which made full recovery difficult. The same phenomenon in general society is many fold worse.

LIFE AFTER THE ARMY

After a total of three years payback to the military for my medical school funding, I followed a romantic interest of mine who was a civilian surgeon to her home city in Ontario. I worked there at a regional cancer centre giving chemo to patients under guidance of medical oncologists, doing cancer research and taking care of very ill patients on the inpatient wards and learning about acute and chronic pain treatment and palliative care from some internationally renowned experts. Amazingly, despite the seemingly depressive work, my "depression" was kept at bay. In fact being in the presence of so many patients who in the face of life-threatening illness displayed such courage, grace and resilience, one could not help but be uplifted, however at a cost of emotional fatigue. Again I found my alcohol use increasing, which was the modus operandi of most of us who spent the most time with the patients: nursing staff, junior doctors and trainees.

I found that the extra energy I felt during internship and residency was kicking in and that the emotional demands were somehow erased by this energy.

I stayed at the cancer clinic for two years. It was here that I met my second wife who was a new grad starting on the cancer inpatient ward. She would put up a lot with my depression as it continued to be misdiagnosed, and the psycho-social upheaval that it caused. Although this relationship lasted ten years, you will see that it came to a tragic end, partly due to her mental health issues, mine and my obsession with my work. This is why from this point I refer to her as 'estranged' although we were married.

During this time I thought that my career path was heading towards medical oncology as a specialist (giving chemo). There was a bureaucratic snag at the time however in that anyone wanting to specialize after having been in practice had no positions available in medical schools to specialize in Canada. What was specifically frustrating was that I had an oncology position at the cancer clinic to do oncology, but I needed to finish my internal medicine specialty before starting it. That's where the problem arose in that no positions were available in Canada for this pre-specialty.

I inquired with the provincial health minister at the time and even confronted the incumbent premier who was seeking re-election. The premier got much negative press for my questioning of him about the specialty after practice issue at a public event and his total inability to answer the question. I still have at least six newspaper clippings sent to me by friends from the entire province lampooning his handling of the issue. I was particularly proud as this premier was a Rhodes Scholar, considered himself to be an academic and went on to be leader of a federal party. Pretty good for a young physician with a history of depression!

NO INTERNAL MEDICINE SPECIALTY PROGRAM IN CANADA FOR ME!

After a few months I did get a position in the United States doing Internal Medicine. If you remember, I said that during my time at the cancer clinic I experienced high energy times despite the rather sombre work subject. About six months into my senior internal medical residency (I had done year one in the military as you recall) in Michigan I again started having symptoms of fatigue, anhedonia (no zest for anything in life), anxiety, poor sleep and decreased libido. It was again a very stressful time in my career, now responsible for junior residents and handling very sick patients, running cardiac arrests, etc. There was also again the issue of twenty-four to thirty-six hour work 'days' and shift work, in general issues that are known to be exacerbating factors for depression.

A Canadian physician who happened to be the Chief of Psychiatry there in the American hospital, prescribed Prozac again (as it had worked previously). However my workload was not stopped entirely and I had to do out-patient internal medicine clinics twice weekly that were considered to be low stress. They usually ran from 10:00 a.m. to 2:00 p.m. I remember being so depressed that I would leave in the morning as if I was going to clinic and then park in a shopping centre parking lot for the duration of "clinic hours", sleep, and then go home. I did this about twice before my excuses were exhausted and I had to bite the bullet and get over my anxieties to return to work.

BACK TO CANADA

Unfortunately, a salary dispute in my final and third year was not remediable even by lawyer intervention and I returned to Canada to practice. (In hindsight, some bipolar type II hypomania may have contributed.) The hospital was offering me a second year salary even though I was to be a final third year resident. I suppose they thought that a polite Canadian would just agree and resume training!

I became extremely busy back in Canada with a full family practice, palliative care and admitting privileges at two city hospitals. I also reviewed internal medicine-related family practice patients for a colleague, half a day a week. Because I was one year short of an internal medicine specialty, I billed this activity as family practice with an interest in internal medicine. I would also cover all the AIDS patients when the local specialist was out of town.

About six months into this hectic schedule, I just woke up one morning and couldn't make myself go to work.

I was intensely fatigued with the depression symptoms already described on several occasions. This time however, I was found to have extremely low levels of testosterone, which were contributing to my fatigue (my now ex-wife and I had also been having problems conceiving). Despite the hormone replacement the symptoms persisted and I was referred to a psychiatrist due to the depth of my depressive symptoms.

My estranged wife endured a great degree of stress at this time. She had to deal with canceling hundreds of patients' appointments, transferring care to other doctors and handling patient queries. In addition we had two mortgages with one house for sale. Physicians have no depression disability insurance so the bills started to pile up. I literally needed prodding to get out of bed each morning content to stay there all day if left on my own. Brushing my teeth was a chore, getting dressed an impossibility. I even had fleeting thoughts of getting into a car while my wife was out, turning on the ignition and leaving the car running in the garage. But they were fleeting.

I went to the psychiatrist faithfully who put me on the old reliable Prozac, which had no effect for over a month. On week five with our life stressors escalating, the psychiatrist tried a hunch. Lithium is a drug that has been used for bipolar disorder for over sixty years. The psychiatrist said that sometimes it can tweak an anti-depressant to start working for simple depression.

THE MIRACLE CALLED LITHIUM

Miraculously, four to five days after going on it I remember waking up to a sunny winter morning with my disposition to match. I felt ready to return to full-time work! After consultation with the psychiatrist however, it was decided that I should return to half-time duties, which was still at least a forty hour work week compared to prior to the depression onset when eighty to ninety was the norm. I returned to work and within months was back to my pre-morbid duties, with *some* decrease in the overall workload, at the suggestion of my psychiatrist.

At no time was any change in my diagnosis made, which is major affective disorder – unipolar – as it was known in those days (depression).

Amazingly, due to my ex-wife and colleagues in the call group I was in (group of doctors that cover for each other in absences), our financial status was stable and my medical practice suffered no irreparable harm from my six to eight weeks of sick leave.

In medicine we say that depression and other mental health disorders are remitting and relapsing, getting better and then coming back. Commonly the reason is the patient stops their medication or never took it properly in the first place (non-compliance). The other unfortunately, is that the physician stops an anti-depressant with resolution of the symptoms, which never should be done in a true diagnosis of depression with very few exceptions. This time my psychiatrist suggested I stay on medications for life.

ONE OF THE FIRST FULL-TIME CANADIAN HOSPITALISTS

The next few years were uneventful. I became one of the first full-time hospitalists in the country. This is a specialist physician that had been present in the United States for years but not prevalent in Canada at the time (see cu*rriculum vitae* link in Appendix 4). Family physicians were and continue to be scarce and most of the family doctors were resigning their positions for following patients while in hospital. Hospitalists directed care and were overall responsible for patients who did not have a family doctor or whose family doctor had no admitting privileges. This ended up being a considerable number. From two of us at the onset of the program, that same hospital now has nine hospitalists, full and part time with ancillary staff. Funnily, my name and the name of the other originating doctor are never mentioned in promotional pieces.[5] The reason for this can be conjectured but I have my own suspicions. The grounds for my opinion become more apparent, I hope, as you read on!

After successfully helping to get this program off the ground, I left following the initial year of the program due to disagreement over compensation. For over six weeks I handled the program on my own due to my colleague's illness. No financial compensation or compensated holiday was offered. After intervention by my legal counsel I was given compensation along with a separation package upon my request. I knew I could not keep up the pace of work demanded by an unappreciative administration (further irony of this sentiment to follow!).

IT'S ALL IN YOUR HEAD!

I left and returned to my hometown where I worked full-time in ER. It was during this stay I developed what sounded like heart pain. Since my dad had his first heart attack at forty-six, my colleagues took it seriously and I went through a dye test of my heart, which showed no blockages, although I required a fair bit of heart medication to give me relief from the pain. The diagnosis could have been one of a controversial condition called Cardiac Syndrome X, or that it was "just in my mind" as I think many of my ER colleagues thought.

However there is a very good body of research that shows that things like depression can bring on cardiac disease[6] and that my depression for which I was on treatment forever, actually did give me heart pain with no real findings. Subsequently the inaccuracy of some health professionals telling patients "it's all in your head" when it really is!

At any rate, the heart pain dissipated and yet again over a dispute of compensation I elected to leave the ER. This time I was working twelve hour shifts in an ER and seeing as many patients as in the regional hospital, which would have up to three doctors working staggered over a twelve hour shift, and I was getting paid fifteen to twenty dollars less per hour. One year later there was a provincial government study of that same ER that suggested increasing the pay to equity with the regional hospital. This ER has now shut down for lack of doctors, and the acute emergency care designation removed from the entire hospital.

I then moved to a very unique position in the near north of Canada working exclusively with First Nations peoples. Our hospital was a secondary care facility with uncomplicated obstetrics, general surgery, mental health counseling, etc. located in Sioux Lookout, a town of about 5000 people in northern Ontario. Each doctor, full and part time, would be responsible for one or several isolated communities in a catchment area larger than France! We were in touch with our communities every day with twenty-four hour coverage by on call doctors overnight, and each of us flying in for one week a month to see patients in our community. A private airline or provincial air ambulance would bring in patients to Sioux Lookout, depending on the urgency of the problem.

My then wife worked full-time in the hospital and we both experienced medicine not otherwise seen down south. The second highest adolescent suicide rate in the world, rickets, tuberculosis, rampant substance dependence and diabetes in up to 60 per cent of certain communities were just *some* of the challenges faced.

Amazingly, I escaped depression while there for a year but had no real psychiatric follow-up for two years, though I faithfully continued all my medication. We left as my wife missed her family in the south and was tiring of the isolation. Despite all the emotional stresses of practice, I found a sense of great solitude in the Sioux with a connection with spirituality that I had never experienced before. This was undoubtedly greatly influenced by the many First Nation friends and culture to which I was exposed.

RACIST UNDERTONES SAW SEVERAL PHYSICIANS OF COLOUR LEAVE

Both my ex-wife as a nurse, and myself as a family doctor with various specialized interests, were avidly recruited in southwest Ontario. We picked a small town close to all my wife's relatives. There was quite a financial incentive to come to the region, but after that, the party was over. There was no help in finding a practice venue, fellow family doctors were standoffish, but at least the specialists were very helpful. As if that was not enough, there were definite racial overtones with patients. For example, over eight physicians of colour left the region within two years of arriving there. Several excuses were made, but the truth was quite apparent in that the need to cope with racism was a large part of their decision to leave.

An illustration of that fact is that up to this time in almost fifteen years of practice I had not received even one complaint against me to any College of Physicians. However in approximately ten years of practice there, I received over ten! This was despite the fact that I had received a *Letter of Commendation* from the Registrar of the College of Physicians and Surgeons of Ontario on being an asset to the medical profession and bringing the art to practice or medicine.

The complaints were incongruent with the commendation, and logic won out, when not even one of the complaints resulted in any disciplinary action against me!

I did however notice that I was becoming increasingly but intermittently irritable with my patients and wife. (This *did* contribute I am sure in some part to the patient complaints albeit no reflection on my knowledge or practice ability.) This culminated with a senseless blow-out one year while on a beach vacation in the Caribbean. I had constant follow-up with my psychiatrist over the ten or so years that we practiced in this small town and was totally compliant with my medication. He also knew about the patient complaints *but said nothing*, especially since they were a very new phenomenon in my relationship with patients.

When I look back in retrospect, my frequent job changes that I thought only meant that I had a wealth of varied experiences, were a more sinister symptom. I was "antsy" often after a few years in a job and had intermittent outbursts of irritability, which were definitely affecting my interpersonal relationships at home and work. As a doctor I knew I was not "manic" in the classic sense, but something was wrong.

TWENTY-FIVE YEARS TO A DEFINITIVE BIPOLAR DIAGNOSIS

I brought this up with my psychiatrist and for the first time in twenty-five years, someone made the connection and diagnosed me as having bipolar type II disorder.

My doctor made some drastic changes in the medications. Within one week I found that my hands were trembling more than usual (small tremor with Lithium was normal), then my writing became illegible. Within two weeks I was having severe difficulties walking up steps. After a few days, walking on the level became awkward. I could no longer practice and had to take a week off work (usually I would be absent only one to two days a year!). I called my psychiatrist who in my opinion flippantly told me that these were only transient side effects (later to be diagnosed as catatonic depression!) and that I should continue with the medications as prescribed.

I became very worried and contacted a medical school buddy of mine who was an academic neurologist in a university setting eighty kilometres away. He graciously saw me quickly with an MRI of the head also being done. Both his exam and the MRI were normal. He suggested side effects from the drugs, but I could tell from his mannerisms (although he had nothing but the most altruistic intentions!) that he thought that the symptoms may indeed be "all in my head", as we have previously discussed.

I told my psychiatrist of the findings and he slowly weaned me off all the new drugs and returned me to the tried and true recipe.

The next six months or so were marked by increasing irritability at work, decreased need for sleep, lessening libido and increasing fatigue. I continued to keep my psychiatrist abreast of what was happening but to no avail. Circumstances were going to dictate a total other path that I would be *forced* to follow.

PHYSICAL ASSAULT ... BY MY WIFE

My former wife came from an extreme of dysfunctional familial backgrounds, filled with a history of substance dependence. She always was a heavy social drinker, but of late it had started to affect her work in my office, her memory, with the addition of alcoholic blackouts. I had counseled both her and her oldest sister that they needed urgent intervention, but in a true example of dependence denial they declined. This was especially frustrating as my wife watched the scourge of substance dependence in my office, many times counseling patients herself!

On May 10, 2010, I returned home late as usual to find my wife in quite an inebriated state. It has to be added that we were dog sitting for her sister's Jack Russell Terrier who terrorized (no pun intended) our four cats and dog. It was always locked up in our bedroom while we were not home and then released in our presence with great caution.

It was on the most trivial of points that my wife started an argument and immediately began to get physical. She did not listen to a word I said and then began pushing me. I avoided any reciprocal contact knowing that the repercussions of a claim of spousal abuse against me, especially in her state of mind would be disastrous *for me*. She then released the Jack Russell from the room and I immediately feared for the welfare of our animals. As I struggled to corral the dog back into a room she began to hit and scratch me chasing the dog and me around the house. I managed to secure the terrier but the onslaught continued with at one point me being pushed into a bathtub and hitting my head. I was dazed for ten or twenty seconds and though bruised, fought my way out of the tub. She blockaded the entrance to the bathroom and I was forced to push my way past with her hitting the floor with no trauma being sustained. I rushed to a portable phone and got only to dial 911 when the phone was hit out of my hand. Luckily the trace on the call summoned police to our address.

My wife was extremely belligerent and abusive to the officers, and a female constable had to be brought in to calm her down. She was shackled and taken down to the police station for booking. The police noted the physical marks on my body and asked that I come down to the police station to give a statement. When I got there, 2:00 a.m. by now, I tried to get the police to drop the charges but they said the Crown had already laid charges of an impaired-related assault charge that could not be retracted. My ex-wife inappropriately called a family friend lawyer and patient as her "one call", which even the police said was improper on the basis of conflict of interest. The lawyer friend apparently visited her in jail that night. (She eventually "fired" him from her case in the ensuing weeks!)

A 500 metre restraining order preventing her contacting me, the house or medical practice was imposed. This effectively ended my relationship with my wife *and* my occupation during a disastrous one hour interaction.

In his late seventies by now, my father, as usual in my corner, flew over 2000 kilometres to be with me the next day. Under police escort my wife removed some personal belongings from the home after being bailed out by her youngest sister, whose husband was a police officer. A bizarre almost psychotic encounter occurred when I saw my soon-to-be ex-sister-in-law. The look in her eyes as my wife obtained some things from the house was beyond one I had ever seen in my mental health patients or even in any Hollywood horror movie. That look is still emblazoned in my mind's eye. The pair secured the belongings they could in fifteen minutes and the restraining order was put in effect.

Over the next few days the enormity of the collapse of my marriage and life's vocation became more and more dire. I pleaded with my father to go to see my wife and talk to her. She had great respect for him as her father was absent from her childhood since she was three years old. He initially said yes but after a night's sleep he reconsidered and said that he did not want to get involved due to her likely unstable mind and the repercussions of him seeing her while I had a restraining order against her. It was a logical argument but one that I did not see in "my state of mind".

TEMPORARY CLOSURE OF MY PRACTICE WITH CLEAR INSTRUCTIONS TO ALL PATIENTS

My father and I had a terrible argument the next morning and in my increasingly disorganized thinking I told him to go home if he was going to be useless. I had a crisis management meeting with the rest of the office staff that evening, and it was decided that they could not cope with the workload without my wife present as she was both the office manager and registered nurse. The conclusion reached at the meeting was that the practice would have to be closed temporarily with patients being given instructions on how they could obtain their medical records. (The local newspaper ran a vindictive story about ten days later about "The Missing Doctor", which was totally inaccurate and libelous, as we did provide instructions to all patients regarding the practice closure.)

With my father gone and the office closed, I felt terribly alone. By this time I was frankly manic, with pressured speech, flight of ideas, disorganized thinking and a distorted view of reality. I had no delusions or hallucinations, but decided to drive two hundred kilometres to where my wife was staying with her youngest sister and husband police officer at 2:00 a.m.; I took along our beautiful dog for the ride, really unsure why.

When I woke everyone up at 3:00 a.m., my brother-in-law came out into the yard and calmly informed me of the danger of my visit with a restraining order in place. I begged that he let me speak with my wife in the yard for only five minutes so that I could plead my case. He finally agreed and my wife came out hesitantly, initially actually asking me how I was doing, but quickly went on the offensive accusing me of having put her in jail and having her experience the most demeaning twelve hours of her life. I stupidly reminded her that it was her actions that had precipitated the entire fiasco and we were off! At the conclusion of the five minutes I asked her if she would consider getting back together, and she said no, but said that she would have to give it some thought. I said little in return and told her I was leaving the dog with her. I hugged and kissed the dog and sped off, now about 4:00 a.m.

GOODBYE

I reached home as the sun began to rise, feeling an eerie peace come over me. The fact that my wife had rejected me, I had lost my occupation (temporarily) and my dog, were as if in another reality. We had three cats at home and I cuddled with each of them. I then gathered heart, blood pressure medication, diabetes pills that I had stolen from my father while he had been there, which as a physician with Internal Medicine training I knew would be a rapid and deadly way of stopping my heart function, lowering my blood pressure and sugar, therefore making resuscitation nearly impossible. I took them with some Scotch and something to make me sleepy in the way of anti-nausea medication. Just before I ingested "the lethal cocktail" I called my wife and said only one word, "Goodbye".

What happened after this is only what has been recounted to me in retrospect, as I was unconscious and on life support for two to three days.

I am told that a police officer neighbour and patient of mine, broke down the door to our home and called 911 when he found me unresponsive. My heart rate was down to thirty beats per minute with no measurable blood pressure. The paramedics who of course I knew personally as well as the ER staff where I worked, did an amazing job of putting intravenouses in my heart to instill blood pressure-raising medications and put me on a breathing machine straight away in the ambulance. Luckily the hospital was only two or three minutes away. My wife was called immediately and a judge lifted the restraining order on compassionate grounds.

Apparently, she and her sister were genuinely upset, crying at my intensive care unit bedside for long periods of time.

A thing used to gauge prognosis in unconscious or coma patients is a type of hand positioning that naturally occurs due to reflexes in the primitive part of the brain. These are known as decorticate and decerebrate posturing and roughly predict long term prognosis.[7]

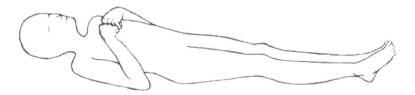

Figure 1 (a) Decorticate posturing.

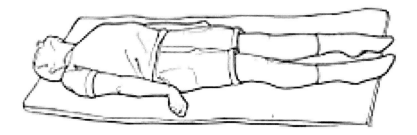

Figure 1 (b) Decerebrate posturing.

I HATE THE COLOUR BLUE FOR A GOOD REASON

Normally people displaying decerebrate or decorticate posturing are in a coma and have poor prognoses, with risks for cardiac arrhythmia or arrest and respiratory failure. The results of decerebrate positioning are usually much more dismal. *This* is what I had, likely due to decreased oxygen to the brain for some period of time.

My wife was asked one of the most difficult questions possible regarding the cessation of my life support due to the poor prognosis. She discussed it with my dad who must have been beyond himself with the sudden news and just having seen me two days before. Lucky for me, the consensus was to continue with the status quo. Miraculously, I started breathing on my own in two to three days and there seemed to be no obvious brain damage. It was excruciating to have well-meaning colleagues come to my step-down ICU bed and question me as to my motives for self-destruction. One in particular was an East Indian physician who had acted as a big brother, which made it particularly difficult. The nurses who all knew me were wonderful under difficult circumstances for them as well, as they were all colleagues of mine in the hospital at the time. The same went for all other members of the health care team especially respiratory therapists who were responsible for my breathing throughout the entire ordeal.

When I was stabilized medically without any complications, I was transferred to a psychiatric facility one hundred kilometres away where my psychiatrist practiced. I could not have stayed in my home hospital since I admitted my own patients there and knew all the staff. However the point is to be made that I had never been on this side of the stethoscope with the psychiatric staff at any hospital!

I was transferred by ambulance by two paramedics I knew well, and who felt equally as awkward as me in having a client who they normally took orders from, but now was a patient restrained on a stretcher five days after a near lethal suicide attempt. It was the first of many awkward experiences that I would experience for a long time.

A family doctor was my first contact on the psychiatric ward after being settled into a semi-private room. His role was to do a medical history and physical. I was put in a blue "Johnny shirt" (a colour I would grow to hate) and pajama bottoms. The doctor accorded me none of the professional courtesy shared by physicians worldwide and seemed to me to be rather condescending. Although I was a patient and he the doctor, I thought it rude that he would interrupt me as I tried to answer a question as best as I could, with the background of a patient who might be able to provide a bit more pertinent medical detail.

After a very superficial exam that would have missed many important findings, especially no neurological exam of note in a patient that had been in a coma, an equally disinterested nurse came in who took a little more psycho-social history, but nothing like what I was used to with our psychiatric nurses in my own hospital or what I expected of myself. It may be said that I was terribly biased in the situation that I was in, but I can honestly say that I was as objective as a person could be in my circumstances.

No psychiatrist met with me for nearly eighteen hours. The next day my own psychiatrist came and rather than being understanding, in my opinion, he admonished me for what I had done. For such a serious clinical turn in my care he only stayed for less than five minutes mainly interested in any suicidal ideation that I may still have. The brevity of the visit was also a harbinger of the "lack of comprehensive care" in mental health that will remain a constant in the rest of my story and sociological commentary.

It was surreal being forced to wear a "blue uniform" (johnny shirt and pajama bottom *ensemble*), street clothes now a privilege held over your head almost mockingly by staff, a sign of trust or form of power over us detainees. The rooms were bare. No window coverings that could be used for self-harm. A single bed sheet and 'blanket' that was more a bed cover than something for warmth. Since it was summer there was only one temperature, cold (air conditioning), more for the staff I'm sure than the patients. The ward consisted of a rectangular ward with a hallway about twenty feet wide that patients were encouraged to walk around and around hundreds of times in a day. This resulted in more anxiety and depression as you constantly met people on your "rounds" talking to themselves or their tormentors, blankly staring off into the distance or looking onto the floor for some lost meaning. (Years later I would become addicted to a television series called *Orange is the New Black*, based on the true story of a New York debutante who was sentenced to 15 months in a minimum security facility ten years after a felony indiscretion. Although the circumstances are certainly different, some of the details of both "incarcerations" are scarily similar!)

Daily psychotherapy by registered nurses or registered practical nurses consisted of five minutes – if you were fortunate enough to have a truly interested nurse – of horribly general questions with no semblance of real therapy as such. If a compassionate person was your guidance for the day, some genuine concern for your present predicament might be expressed, but almost never in my entire hospital stay was a true psychotherapy session given. This was partly due to the fact that nurses said they didn't have enough time, but if you observed the time they socialized, the latter was not the case.

Now let me make it clear. There were a *handful* of nurses that came to their very difficult job every day with the aim to help patients. I was very fortunate to have these nurses when they were too seldom randomly assigned to me. Their faces and voices would *temporarily* bring a ray of light onto a chronic cloudy day. Their words not having anything to do with psychotherapy were comforting, and they would not let me slack off on my daily hygiene or self-care. At the end of their shift I knew that someone had taken care of me that day with concern in their heart or soul, with empathy, not sympathy.

AN ANGEL OF A HOUSEKEEPER

Probably one of the most genuinely interested staff was a housekeeper who every day drew a sun, rainbow or flower on our orientation board, which was *supposed* to have the day of the week and date on it as we had no calendars, watches, cell phones, etc. The orientation portion was almost never up to date and was to be changed each day by your nurses to inform you of whose charge you were each day. I will never forget that housekeeper's kindness. Her heartfelt queries about how I was progressing, if I had received any visitors, did I enjoy my meal that day, etc. were a highlight of my banal existence. At the end of my stay she gifted me a bookmark that I cherish to this day, one of the few photographs in this book.

'NUTRITIOUS DIET' WAS AN OXYMORON

Speaking of meals, there was a rotated menu week after week. It was often not even geared to your medical condition, that is morbidly obese patients getting two meals if there were extras, along with leftover desserts, or diabetics – of which probably one-third of the patients were – receiving a normal diet. Another major issue were nightly snacks, which consisted of bread, jam, butter/margarine, peanut butter, scant fruit of poor quality and highly sugared fruit juice with preservatives. At 8:00 p.m. each night there would literally be a stampede of patients towards the trough, with jam and juice gone within seconds. Again, no medical attention was paid to sugar control in diabetics or type and portion amount in obese patients. The majority of patients, at least 70 per cent, were obese and/or diabetic as per the following.

In fact studies released just about the time of my admission to hospital revealed the facts about a condition known as 'metabolic syndrome' in mental health patients:

Metabolic syndrome appears increased in patients with severe mental illness
Based on a cross-sectional study in Australia

203 patients aged 18-65 years with schizophrenia, schizoaffective disorder, bipolar disorder, major depressive disorder with psychotic symptoms, drug-induced psychosis or borderline personality disorder were evaluated for metabolic syndrome

Prevalence of metabolic syndrome:

54% in all patients
67% in patients with bipolar disorder
67% in patients with schizoaffective disorder
51% in patients with schizophrenia[8]

In short, a person with this syndrome is *twice* as likely to develop heart disease[I] and *five times* as likely to develop diabetes[II] as someone who doesn't have metabolic syndrome.

I   The consequences are astounding! If you consider that currently 1 in 4 Canadians die of cancer and 1 in 3 die of heart attack or stroke, the *majority* of people with significant mental health issues (millions in Canada) have a *two in three chance* to have or die from heart disease (2 x 1/3).

II   Public Health Agency of Canada. *Diabetes in Canada: Facts and Figures from a Public Health Perspective.* (Ottawa, 2011). Accessed June 7, 2015. www.phac-aspc.gc.ca/cd-mc/publications/diabetes-diabete/facts-figures-faits-chiffres-2011/highlights-saillants-eng.php#chp1.

A very common side effect of many mental health drugs is the development of diabetes mellitus (DM), whether it be from medications for bipolar depression or schizophrenia. According to the Public Health Agency of Canada, in 2008/09 some 6.8 per cent of Canadians were living with DM, with another 20 per cent undiagnosed. DM is the fastest growing disease in Canada, with 60,000 new cases a year. Mental health patients have a 34 per cent *or 1 in 3 chance of developing DM (6.8 x 5 times risk; extrapolating from the above Australian data)*, not accounting for the fact that many psychotropics (psychiatric drugs) cause DM.

If you have DM, your risk for heart attack or stroke is also increased. Many of the hundreds of patients I saw while an inpatient in the hospital were not even assessed for this crippling untreated disease *or* metabolic syndrome, because statistically I should have seen them being diagnosed and put on appropriate diets as documented in the Australian study of 2009. I was in hospital for a total of *fifteen months*, with only brief *disastrously* short, intervening premature discharges and readmissions!

The sheer irony is that over the length of my admission I would lose about *thirty kilograms (about seventy pounds)* from psychiatric illness(decreased appetite), improper caloric supplementation and neglect of my complex medical condition.

Now the sheer length of time of my admission is not only rare but was one of the longest that any patient had incurred in that hospital's psychiatric ward history. This simple fact raises the inefficiency of care that was provided to a physician (me) who could clearly present his history and clinical progress, but on average had two-minute psychiatrist visits daily over a year and a quarter, maybe five-minute nurse "psychotherapy" sessions per day and so-called occupational therapy (OT) daily

This OT was provided by two well-meaning therapists, only one of whom was a trained OT. The ineffectiveness of OT treatment however, was due to the system not providing the therapist with enough money to design effective treatment plans and the fact that they would be overwhelmed in performing their tasks effectively. The therapists even spent their own money to provide art supplies, etc. for the limited therapy that they could administer.

A hospital inpatient OT program is supposed to provide patients with practical life skills that can be used upon discharge; for mental health patients skills such as so-called activities of daily living (ADLs) – socialization skills, shopping, money management, cooking, personal hygiene and grooming, *medication compliance*, use of walking aids and general coping skills for practical everyday life, etc. The only therapy we had was colouring with coloured pencils/crayons, painting with oil paints and water colours, playing video games and other useless therapy games. The honest truth was that the nursing staff *pushed* all patients regardless of degree of socialization ability, sedation, anxiety and depth of depression to mandatory participation.

Mandatory OT participation meant that nurses and ward staff had ninety minutes time off daily, as I overheard several nurses say during my residence on the psychiatric ward when they thought I was not hearing. In fact I would overhear many other things that would be rather astounding over my stay. A large amount of time was spent by nursing staff discussing personal events behind the desk. When a patient came to the desk they were often asked to wait twenty minutes to half an hour while you heard your nurse discussing recipes or extracurricular activities of their kids. The ward clerks were so rude that they would not even acknowledge your presence standing there in front of them for five to ten minutes at a time. They would not even be talking to a nurse or on the phone, but would just keep you waiting in a deliberate show of false authority or genuine meanness. At other times they too were heard talking on the phone about personal "stuff" or family matters while we waited for a medication, a treatment question, keys to get a shower/asking for towels or sometimes just to have water jugs filled. The drugs used to treat depression often cause severe dry mouth.

The OT was therefore useless for any rehabilitative purposes. Mental health patients require immense life skill training, which is certainly not found during hospital stays and is non-existent in group homes. These homes are very often where patients are transferred post-discharge, some because they need constant supervision, some because they have no home. These are mostly funded to line the pockets of the home operators. They are rotating repositories of partially-treated patients and at times patients who have not recovered at all but were discharged from hospital due a lack of beds.

The non-compliance rate with mental health patients and medications is a huge problem as already mentioned and varies from study to study and specific illnesses considered. Some schizophrenia estimates and those with bipolar patients say that over 50 per cent of these mental health patients stop using their medications for reasons of side effects, "feeling better" or just not remembering to take them.

A comprehensive OT and social work (SW) treatment plan would work wonders in preventing readmission to hospital and supporting compliance. Social workers during my stay were quite negative in their view of my illness. Focus on how to get discharged and not on why I was there. One of my greatest problems was getting back together with my wife, as unhealthy as that may have been. However one SW simply repetitively told me "to get on with my life", when my reputation, marriage and ostensibly my career were all gone.

During my fifteen months in hospital, my estranged wife neglected to arrange to have my medical licence renewed, failed to pay on several credit cards, did not pay any income tax for my personal account and joint corporation for two years (which she normally did for our corporation and two personal tax accounts) and according to my divorce legal counsel embezzled some $450,000 CDN over the course of our marriage. (She was found to have a secret bank account during the legal discovery process!)

Both the SW and my psychiatrist did not provide me with any advice for handling these gargantuan issues, which would affect anyone's life, let alone someone admitted for refractory depression for over a year!

Things were to get much worse believe it or not.

After three weeks of admission my psychiatrist deemed me fit for discharge. This was despite the fact that the night before being let go

I was warned about fraternizing with female patients. Hypersexuality is a well-known symptom of mania and I even recognized that I was still a bit high like I had been at the time of my suicide attempt. But that same realization made me think I was all right for discharge, like an impaired driver thinking that they are fit to drive.

I was discharged home and took the train, being so inattentive as to lose one bag with my wallet and all my ID, which should have been a sign of things to come.

I arrived in my driveway with a next door neighbour greeting me at the door. She was a patient of mine along with her ten-year-old son and undoubtedly had seen the parade of emergency vehicles around the house recently. She was a good friend of my estranged wife and how much she knew of the dramatic events that had ensued is unknown. It is my suspicion that my wife, if not then but assuredly later, had spun a tail recounting the events in her favour, with the neighbours aware of her arrest and charges through the neighbourhood police officer. The neighbour was also acquaintances with the policeman who had saved my life. His wife was a bit of a gossip and had likely informed this neighbour of what had gone on if my wife had not. I also was the family doctor to this police officer, his wife and two daughters.

The neighbour was quite friendly as I recall through a manic haze and I invited her over as it seemed the correct thing to do since she seemed to be so supportive. She came over with a soft drink without hesitation and we sat on the recreation room couch with at least two feet separating us. The unusual thing with mania is that you remember events but behaviour remains to some extent out of your control. *She* asked to go to look at the basement that had recently been totally redone due to mold. She had discussed this project in detail with my wife as the gutting and rebuilding had occurred. We went down to the basement and looked at reconstruction for five minutes then went upstairs back to the recreation room.

She was still drinking her soft drink. As I already mentioned I was her family doctor. I knew from conversations with my wife that she and her husband had longstanding marital issues. In my hypomanic and hypersexual state I asked her questions about her marriage that I normally would not have addressed. *They were not at all provocative.* Equally as unusual, I put my hand on her knee while we were speaking, but *not* associated with any sexual overtones either verbally or with any gesture.

I remember that she became uncomfortable and calmly made an excuse to leave and I accompanied her to the front door. She had crossed to her yard across a fence and inexplicably, I pulled down my pants as we saw each other again from the confines of our yards separated by a fence and approximately 150 yards. Again I emphasize that in a hypomanic or manic state one cannot control your behaviour although you may have perfect recollection of the event. The neighbour did not scream or make an emergent gestures, but I lost sight of her as I went back into the house, locked the door and went into a deep sleep on the couch where we had been sitting.

I must have been asleep for a couple of hours when I heard a sudden loud knock on the door. I was still too asleep and hypomanic to open the door, but finally I went over to it and opened it slightly to see who it was. Even in the throes of hypomania I still half knew who it might be. Two municipal policemen presented themselves and said that I was under arrest for some charge to this day I don't recall. I went with them without complications in a pair of shorts, golf shirt and sandals. I was put in a cell, given booties instead of my sandals and my watch was taken from me.

I fell asleep right away on the metal bench and at about 2:00 a.m. according to the wall clocks, was fingerprinted and photographed. It was at this time I was charged with sexual harassment. I was extremely cold I remember and was given a space blanket. The next morning I was given a fast food coffee and breakfast sandwich. A point to know is that I had at least six municipal policemen/provincial police officers and their families in my practice. I am sure that the news of my arrest *flew* through the law enforcement community. I also had a few prominent lawyers and civic officials as patients, which made things worse. Also many prominent business persons and socialites in the community would have known in short order in a town of thirty thousand inhabitants.

The police officer who had rescued me during my suicide attempt visited along with another officer (my patient) who was assigned to take me back to the psychiatric ward after the arraignment. Both showed indifference. I appeared via camera in front of the judge who explained the charges of sexual assault and appointment of a defence counsel by the court. Present was yet another police officer patient of mine. I agreed to everything, signed on the dotted line as instructed and was given a court date.

I was put into a police car with metal handcuffs behind my back with my patient police officer and his partner. We started on our one hour journey. I slept again for most of the trip but was awakened by the cuffs digging into my wrists. My "patient officer" was kind enough to pull over onto the shoulder on Canada's busiest highway and loosen the cuffs.

We arrived at the hospital having to go through the ER where again I knew most of the staff and had worked for several years, and was back on the ward less than twenty-four hours after being discharged! The nurses were anything but sympathetic and actually quite condemning in my eyes, assuming my guilt before a judgement was done. I guess I was still quite hyper, and totally not recalling the circumstances, was transferred to the PICU (psychiatric intensive care unit). This unit is reserved for violent and uncooperative patients but very often over my fifteen month stay was noted to house patients with no strict admission criteria. I certainly was not any of the aforementioned, but may have been a bit talkative.

The PICU consisted of a super lockdown unit (all psychiatric wards were locked but this ward much more so). There were rooms with no doors but a few rooms with one foot thick, wood doors with a space to push in a dinner tray at the bottom. At the top was a one by one foot heavily reinforced window with poor visibility of the entire room. There were however cameras in each isolation room for observation at the nursing station. I vividly remember being put in the PICU and allowed to walk about freely. There was an older female nurse at the desk and I remember asking for a glass of water. She rudely answered that she was busy and that I should come back. I came back about fifteen minutes later and inexplicably I was suddenly grabbed by two male nurses one at my hands and the other at my feet. I understandably struggled but they overpowered me and just as I was being put in the isolation room I recall slamming the back of my head very hard on the tile floor with likely concrete underneath (I assume so, as I developed shin splints from doing miles and miles of rounds of walking in the ward on this same floor).

No attention was given to my complaint.

These two male nurses and the older female RN came back in short order and I was forcibly given a shot in my buttock. The rest is a blur.

I do recall that all there was in my "cell" was a mattress on the floor. Only when the drugs had worn off did I realize that there was a bathroom in the room. In the absence of that I relieved myself of urine on the floor while lying down and drank it. I was too sedated to eat any of the food slid into the room because I couldn't stand because of the drugging. (This is all reminiscent of anything I have seen or heard about solitary confinement units in prison, only in this case meant for *sick patients* and not for criminals. A declaration from the United Nations shows that some of the confinement practices in prison are inhumane and contrary to human rights codes worldwide.)

What I do remember is that subconsciously, I convinced myself that I could not move due to my head trauma (half being in a drug-induced stupor with faulty reasoning and half recalling something of being a "doctor"). The nurses were singularly unsympathetic but someone must have taken this seriously. I was taken restrained to either a CT or MRI scan of my brain. I would have a couple more of these during my stay.

I am unsure how long I actually stayed in lockdown or more importantly *why* in the first place. I was never violent, uncooperative or refused medication. To this day I wonder if it was retribution for the fact that I had committed a *putative* crime while being *prematurely* discharged from hospital of no accord of my own! At any rate I was released to a no-door bed in the PICU after my solitary confinement. The medication must have been lowered because I now was aware of my surroundings, saw where I had been locked up (discovered there indeed was a bathroom, although I had been physically incapable of using it) and started to recall more of what had gone on "during my time away".

I was eventually discharged back to the *normal* ward.

Life on this ward was interminable. Soon the highs of hypomania were replaced by a depression not comprehensible to anyone who has not experienced it. Imagine the saddest you have ever felt, the least amount of energy that you have ever had, the smallest bit of hope you have ever had and the least desire to live that you have experienced. Then, multiply that by a thousand, or ten thousand or even a million. That's the only way I can describe depression but even that is inadequate.

Best-selling author William Styron, in his candid account of his battle with depression, puts it much more eloquently:

> *The pain of severe depression is quite unimaginable to those who have not suffered it, and it kills in many instances because its anguish can no longer be borne. The prevention of many suicides will continue to be hindered until there is a general awareness of the nature of this pain.*[9]

You rue each day as you wake up because the misery begins. Only sleep provides refuge as your brain stops and peace can temporarily ensue. You have no appetite. You need sleeping pills to provoke you into that state of heaven each night.

You don't want to talk to anyone. Staying literally covered to the head in your sheets all day is the definition of *waking* hell. You are surrounded by people with the same misery or worse. People talking to themselves as they walk hundreds of times around the halls, very loud patients discussing absurdities with other patients or out and out fights, and verbal or otherwise struggles between patients-patients or patients-staff.

In my case it was made much worse as often some of my own patients from the past were admitted and recognized me. I would force out a perfunctory "Hi" then disappear into my room.

I always had a roommate who inevitably slept all day (hundreds through *fifteen months*), which was fine by me as stellar conversation was not even a dream in my condition. The nurses would drag you out of the safety of your room to shower each day in common showers for up to fifty people. I noted that these were never disinfected even after ten showers and sometimes not for two days in a row. Mental health patients by the nature of their disease have very poor hygiene. Many I noticed had infected sores from self-scratching, foot conditions visible in flip-flops that even made me a physician of twenty years look away, and the smell of intertrigo (yeast growing in folds of obese people; maybe 50 per cent of patients on the ward conservatively) was as common as food smells at mealtime. I had an aversion to showering due to a fear of catching some infection. I would soon learn how dangerous for me this would have been.

I *luckily* had moderate to severe psoriasis (for which I had been on study drugs and gave side effects very similar to chemotherapy and even chances of cancer from the drug itself). My disease flared almost throughout the admission and at one point was so unmanageable that I had to go to my specialist with a nurse escort. In an incredible stroke of luck that contributed to my overall *happiness*, the specialist had hired my ex-wife and refused to treat me on the grounds of conflict of interest. In retrospect this was against ethical rules of medical practice, but in my condition I was in no place to argue. This dermatologist continues to be more interested in making money from very lucrative medical trials than the average of two to three minutes per regular patient as verifiable by anyone that has seen him. In addition, though I had long been a colleague, I was now presenting as a psychiatric, suicidal inpatient.

This dermatologist had given up his hospital privileges years ago due to the lack of remuneration for hospital work, as he himself once told me when I was a full-time hospitalist.

So for most of my stay I suffered from up to 25 per cent body surface area, severely itchy, scaling skin and occasional bleeding from excessive scratching. This is why I say I was *lucky* because I had a very plausible medical excuse for not showering every day due to the drying effect on the psoriasis. I was never provided with any up to date drugs for the condition, only topical steroids, which have many known side effects used over a long period of time.

This brings me to another related issue. All the doctors but one seeing me for medical and non-psychiatric problems were members of my old call group, that is one in every five weekends one physician would take care of the entire group's patients in two hospitals. This required much trust in one another, and I even took one of the physicians as my doctor and I, her husband, as mine. I also provided the group advice at their asking on some of my interests such as chronic pain, palliative care and some internal medicine issues. As previously said, one of the group was the only "AIDS doc" in the area at a time when there were no infectious disease specialists. Although a family doctor, he amazingly trained himself with conferences, reading, seminars, etc. to treat what at the time was a deadly and extremely complex disease that today is totally different. He trusted me with taking care of this huge in and out patient practice in his absence. This same physician does not even acknowledge me since my recovery three years later, even while we are in a patient room for whom I am advocating.

None of these physicians took more than two minutes to speak with me during my fifteen month hospitalization, treating me as a medical problem in a psychiatric patient and not once asking how I felt or even showing compassion for a former colleague. I suppose this was the "professional" thing to do, but it certainly was not the compassionate. In fact they should have signed off my case for lack of objectivity, which as we will see soon, resulted in disastrous medical consequences for me.

Almost three months went by and despite several medicine changes my mood stayed as dismal as it had been. If possible the days got greyer. I had no visitors outside my estranged wife who continually harassed me, until even my psychiatrist restricted visits for signatures for business purposes only. I constantly still wanted her back, which in my depressed state I thought might lead to some return to normalcy. Little did I realize that she was systematically destroying my profession, finances, reputation and savings. While doing this, she took up romantically with a pharmaceutical representative that had visited my office for over ten years with her present. He was at least twenty years her senior and her numerous absences of six to eight hours shopping on Saturdays (over the last two to three years of our marriage) while I was at work or resting, now made sense. He lived forty-five minutes from our marital home. My ex-wife had already admitted to a one night stand in year five of our marriage.

My depression was stagnant with no action on my psychiatrist's part to change treatment. In fact he would go on one week absences/holidays more frequently as my hospitalization progressed, which made me wonder if he was healthy. The negative side for me was that over likely *eight weeks* of my *fifteen month* stay he was not there, and patient-sitting, stand-in psychiatrists made no treatment changes during these absences leaving the *status quo* of my refractory (treatment-resistant in doctor talk) depression.

As the weeks went by I realized that my lifelong passion was in jeopardy, *the College had revoked my licence to practice medicine due to application non-renewal.* My estranged spouse did not bring the forms to me and I was not mentally competent to complete the application at any rate. She could have notified the College and so could have my psychiatrist, but neither was done.

She did not pay *three* credit cards over *fifteen* months and did not submit the corporation (medical practice) or my personal taxes to our accountant, knowing I was incapable and more importantly, as she had done regularly over ten years of marriage.

As previously mentioned, she also had a secret bank account where a forensic auditor concluded she had embezzled plus or minus $450,000 CDN with the help of an accountant. Lastly, although she did sell the matrimonial home (money in her pocket) she left the office building belonging to our joint corporation unoccupied but still being paid for by myself with no income. I would later receive $100,000 CDN for a reason that I would have rather not had, but she too managed this money, with me medically incompetent for financial and personal care decisions in hospital for fifteen months.

Repeated meetings with my social worker regarding these life crises only resulted in the *sage* advice that, "Alcoholics shouldn't marry bipolar patients", and that, "Your wife is an evil person from whom you should stay away!" This of course had the expected effect of worsening my depression and causing me to have a totally bleak outlook for the future even if I recovered.

The most activity that I saw from this social worker was when he absconded with the patient copy of the newspaper almost daily and spent an hour at least behind the nursing station catching up on the day's events. The newspaper usually would not be returned to its rightful owners!

By that time, maybe five or six months into my stay, I was given the great privilege of my own clothes (not really mine, but graciously given to me by the hospital women's auxiliary charity drives, as my wife had brought me nothing but a wallet). Along with this came the luxury of smoke breaks (which approximately 75 per cent of patients attended) or walking on the hospital grounds for short periods, the exact duration of which I do not recall. The walks added little to someone who still found it uncomfortable to leave their room. Again, if you have never experienced the depths, it's hard to relate. I stayed in hospital gowns because I couldn't summon up the energy or will to change most days.

I did however start reading everything in sight, interacting with the other patients mostly in their untreated state was impossible. Of no fault of their own, my fellow *inmates* were argumentative, loud, sometime verbally abusive or manifesting other symptoms of their disease that made social interaction difficult. At that time talking with somebody on the outside was even difficult with my rejection of calls from my father weekly. He dutifully called every Sunday to try and speak with me but I refused, leaving him to get an update from the nurses. The nurses chastised me and tried to make me feel guilty about my dad, but in that depth of depression you don't care about anybody or anything.

The one TV was at least ten years old, normally monopolized for trashy reality shows where infidelity was treated as a game show and whooping from the studio audience and the patient audience unbearable. Even staff sat in to watch. I tried to view the news, sports or other more cerebral shows but was almost always voted down. I would therefore retreat to my room, get under the covers and read, the only place that one really feels safe in any more than a mild depressive state. Board games, cards and other distractions were again old and incomplete, with no one really able to play because of acute treatment or their illness, with decreased attention spans, patience and recall.

A very sad occurrence for me involved the only *TV buddy* I met in my fifteen month stay. He on the surface was a very controlled schizophrenia patient who was admitted several times, never for overtly psychotic episodes, but I am presuming an inability to take care of himself, or someone noting early that he was coming off his meds. He was a tall (6 feet, 3 inches at least) lanky fellow, with his outstanding feature a bushy, long black beard, something you would imagine the Québécois lumberjacks of legend to sport. He would spend ninety per cent of his time making endless rounds of the ward with a military-like precise cadence only stopping for water, meals or the odd break. However, the exception was sports on TV. This was when I had an ally in wanting to watch something on TV, outvoting the reality TV junkies.

We watched Sunday afternoon football, hockey and I especially remember one World Series. He would get up to walk between innings, at half-time or between periods for a round of the ward. We would share *short* comments on plays, as socialization is not a forte in schizophrenia especially in his medicated state (and my general anhedonia). We showed no emotion at exciting plays or touchdowns, home runs or goals. Every time he was readmitted I would still be there and we would watch the sport in season. Strangely, no one challenged us during our prolonged watching sessions, and even the nurses extended curfew hours for special sporting events. He even shaved his beard the last time I saw him which made him look so young.

One day, while I was not better feeling better at all at about month seven to eight, I heard he had committed suicide. It was devastating especially because I wished that it was *me instead of him.*

The suddenness of the news, heartbreak of the premature and senseless loss of such a young, gentle giant (one of the nurses said he was twenty-four years old) did cause me great *hurt for him* and even further dejection

Unfortunately another very quiet and pleasant lady with young kids that I knew less well, also jumped into the icy river that flanks the northern part of our city, her body recovered days later. In all there were at least two other suicides by people who had been on the ward while I was admitted over the fifteen months.

As I mentioned, I read voraciously. When finished the "ward library" some nurses who were among the most considerate, albeit of little true therapeutic assistance, brought books from home for me to read. I usually finished a book a day, but faithfully this dedicated book brigade managed to find me mostly mystery and suspense novels to read for three to five months. By then I had pretty much depleted their respective collections.

Shortly after the suicide of my friend, I was dealt a blow, that is a stay of charges that would be requested in my *assault* case necessitated that I appear in court in my hometown to enter a plea in person. I walked several times to the office of one of the best criminal attorneys in the province and perhaps country, a six to seven kilometre round trip, on special passes. We discussed a plea of innocent due to mental health issues with no permanent record unless I offended again within a year, that is a stay of charges.

The lawyer was exceedingly kind and sympathetic to my situation. He even picked me up at the hospital and drove me to my hometown for the court appearance. As I had dreaded, I met patients of mine who even sitting directly behind me in the court waiting room, did not acknowledge me. This one patient was a twenty-year-old mother of three children ranging from one year to three and a half. I had gone out of my way to help her, even getting her out of a brutal child abuse situation with one of the fathers. Not a nod.

More interestingly was the absolute ignorance of the police officer/neighbour who had saved my life during my initial suicide attempted. As earlier mentioned, I had taken care of three generations of his family and done several favours for them. His only comment was, "I have nothing to say to you because you sexually assaulted..." No queries as to the possible circumstances, my story (which he should have elucidated as an active detective constable) or giving me the benefit of a doubt with all the things I had done for his family (including several house calls!).

The hearing itself was quick and sweet. While my lawyer was with the judge I ran into my business lawyer in the waiting area, whose daughter I ironically admitted to psychiatry and stabilized years earlier for bipolar disorder. I took care of three generations of his family including his in-laws. I preferentially gave help to his mother who had terrible heart disease until the time of her death.

He couldn't get away from me fast enough in my opinion. I inquired of his family. He had been the one my ex-wife had hired the night of her arrest but had since fired. Had he been able to pull a cloak of invisibility around him he may have felt better.

The hearing went well, and my lawyer was to appear without my appearance in six months. On the way home I was honoured that a person of such prominence opened up to me about his family. For about one hour he sought my advice as to whether one of his sons may have mental health disease. A very bizarre occurrence for a lawyer driving a doctor home from a criminal charge plea on the basis of mental health extenuating circumstances. He was profoundly and eons ahead of the societal stigma associated with mental health, partly because of his family situation and partly due to the thousands of mental health patients he had defended in his career. Not only did he take my advice, but at the end of our dealings together he returned a significant portion of my retainer!

AFTER ONE YEAR MY CHARGES WERE STAYED!

Ultimately, my *charges were stayed* and *removed from the books* one year after the plea, without *any* legal consequences, *but* a partially libellous story *stays online* that affects me to this day in almost every aspect of my life.

A break in the monotony I didn't expect was one day when I was approached by the staff psychometrist. (A psychometrist is responsible for the administration and scoring psychological and neuropsychological tests under the supervision of a clinical psychologist or clinical neuropsychologist. Psychometrist training should have an emphasis on accuracy, validity, and standardization in administration.) Their work can add to the diagnosis of a psychiatrist showing abnormalities that may not be noted on CT or MRI scans for example head trauma, drug-use brain damage, birth-related problems, etc. The results sometimes are affected by organic illness such bipolar disorder and schizophrenia, so that careful analysis for confounding variables must be studied.

The test is so grueling that it must be done over two days or more due to patient fatigue. It measures reading, comprehension, 3D conception and planning and many other variables of which I was not even aware. My results were very interesting. They showed that I had changes on one side of my brain with slight comprehension and visualization deficit, not enough to affect my ability to practice medicine however. The conjecture was that the changes may be from head trauma. I never really had any significant trauma in playing sports for years, having played a lot of ice hockey and soccer, but did have a history of *having been dropped recently on my head!* The clinical psychologist said that the changes could have been from that incident but also from my bipolar disorder acutely. I have never had the tests repeated due to lack of access to the clinical psychologist and psychometrist.

If I seem to be very critical or even a little vindictive, it was because a lot of things were going wrong in my epic stay. By six months, little or nothing had changed. My mood was in the doldrums, my worries over a career I had built over twenty years, financial issues and my personal life had as much hope and light as six months of darkness in Nunavut.

You have to remember that I was a physician who on the books had had twenty-eight hundred patients (on paper), in a thriving Family Practice with interest in Internal Medicine, Chronic Pain and Palliative Care. I was used to working eighty hours per week including weekends and traveling the world every three months, all snatched away from me in one horrible night.

I therefore decided to take issues into my own hands, still in a cavernous depression, but almost equaled by an overwhelming feeling that my entire life was crumbling down around me, and that no one cared. Desperation is another word that came to mind.

I was still in possession of my daily breaks on outside grounds. One fall night I went out on an evening break and didn't come back. In total control of my faculties but still deeply depressed – there is a major difference, with the latter causing abnormal and uncontrollable behaviour due to the disease – I decided to catch a bus 100 kilometres to my home where my wife now had legal permission to live while I was not there (restraining order lifted due to my hospitalization). Her charges were still waiting to be addressed in court.

Despite all that had been told to me by the social workers and psychiatrist about the unsuitability of an ongoing relationship with my estranged wife, my desperate thinking dictated the logic that getting back together with her could restore my practice and finances. In addition, anyone with even mild to moderate/severe depression will tell you that one yearns for affection. My family were on the other side of the country and I had shut them out. She was the only source of affection or caring I *thought* I had. Again using the word desperation multiple times, I extended my hand out for help.

When I arrived at the house, she was ice cold, still spouting abusive anger about *my* getting *her* arrested and charged. (At any point I could have made her College of Nurses aware of the alcoholism and criminal charges. No one did, especially me who had suffered so much at her hands.) *I*, admitted for almost a year and a half on a psychiatric ward directly due to her actions, my entire world in tatters, pleaded for another chance. It was rejected in a cruel manner.

I did notice that she was trying to rush me out of the house continually. She mentioned that the hospital ward had called asking about my whereabouts, but she had made no effort to call them back, funnily, to tell them of my location. She also did not want to call police. She did give me minutes to be with my dog and four cats, none of whom recognized me after nearly a six month absence. But still, she literally physically ushered me out the door, albeit with the keys to a car that was rightfully mine. What she thought I should do with a car as a hospital inpatient I am to this day unsure.

The key chain had the key to my office building which was still on the real estate market, and for which *I* was paying the mortgage as a hospital inpatient.

My spouse was a legal partner in the corporation responsible for the property as previously mentioned.

ANOTHER SUICIDE ATTEMPT

Feeling yet *another* defeat in a life of now no wins, I lost to impulsiveness found often in bipolar disorder. As I mentioned earlier, one of my clinical interests was treatment of chronic pain. This meant that my office had a huge cache of very strong narcotic pain killers, which taken in high enough doses cause cessation of breathing. I had an expert's knowledge of the use of these pills.

One doesn't really think of what you're doing at times like this. It's that proverbial "I was looking from above down on me" experience. I calculated the dosage to be enough to acutely kill me with quick-acting drugs, then just to make things interesting I added a huge dose of long-acting narcotic that would stay in my system for weeks should I survive the initial onslaught. Either way, I would relieve myself of the conscious hell that I was living.

I then drove the car to an isolated country lane about twenty kilometres out of town and crashed the car into a water-filled ditch. I received no injury that I recall. It was fall in Canada. As the frigid water filled the car I was rudely awoken to my reality. I called 911.

The answering police officers upon arrival asked me what I had done and if I had attempted it before. Upon my answering yes, the attitude of all four-five officers on scene changed to one of derision.

"Why do you keeping on doing this, and you're a doctor?" Their question was answered by no response as I lost consciousness. In retrospect, with my cynicism today, I should have answered, "It's my hobby!"

I awoke again in the ICU, my spouse who lived five minutes away never to be present over my five to seven day admission. I was on a ventilator for days as any attempt to wean me off resulted in my breathing becoming critical.

Normally when we encounter an unconscious patient in the ER, it is a reflex to administer glucose (sugar low as in a diabetic), a drug called Naloxone (*instantly* reverses narcotic effect if the blood levels are not extremely high, sub lethal or lethal) and Flumazenil (slowly reverses effects of certain types of anxiety or sleeping pills called benzodiazepines). In my case because the blood levels of narcotics were so high (as I had calculated) the doctors had to consult a university centre and start me on a Naloxone drip that was dripping into my veins twenty-four hours daily. With that change, I was able to come off the breathing machine days later but still needed quite a bit of oxygen.

Every time a small drop in the Naloxone was attempted, I went into a feeling that with even what was to happen with me later on, was the most horrible sensation ever. It was literally as if someone was standing on your lungs and you couldn't move them in or out (*a reminder of how my mom must have felt when she was dying*), and my oxygen levels would drop dangerously low in seconds. Even in severe asthma there is some air movement though it may be little air movement. The result can be fatal in acute asthma unless proper treatment is quickly administered and the severity of the attack recognized. It even came to the point that I would uncontrollably spit during one of these several drug-weaning attempts of struggling to get a breath, obviously upsetting the nurses (who ended up recipients of projection saliva) who for the most part were stellar and most of whom I known professionally as previously stated.

Still on a Naloxone drip, (the university hospital that was consulted, at this point had never seen someone on this route of medication as long; I guess my dose calculations had been correct) it was eventually decided that although I was not stable medically, I be transferred to the hospital from which I had *escaped*, so that I may stay in their ICU and still be seen by my psychiatrist.

I dreaded the prospect of returning to that *prison* devoid of hope.

An ambulance with an ICU RN escort due to my fragile medical status was used for transporting me back to the place I dreaded. In the ICU of my hospital admission, the attitude of staff was again anything but understanding, with the very real sentiment expressed by the attending physician that I was occupying a much needed bed. The nurses may have been a little less harsh, but not by much. Over a total of four or five days (including time spent in the last ICU), the Naloxone drip was stopped and I was carefully watched for any breathing problems. My psychiatrist only visited once over this time and was angry at me for a second suicide attempt and had little more to add, not even a query about what desperation had driven me once again to this action. He seemed to be more interested in the fact that my absconding from hospital had put *him* in a medico-legal situation.

As I recovered I oddly found myself wishing that I would become more ill so as to stay in the ICU and avoid returning to the *hole*. However, the day finally arrived and it was back to the hell that I had experienced for about one half year to date, my mood now worse, with feelings of guilt about the second suicide attempt, not treated by anyone as a worsening of my mental health. No change in medication was administered, though the nurses were somewhat more forgiving of my act.

The *status quo* returned to normal with me camping out under my covers exhausting the world's supply of mystery/suspense novels. The habit of no psychotherapy and occupational therapy of little use ensued, and of course my social worker just had an "I told you so" message about having approached my soon to be ex-wife. (The newspaper still disappeared from the patient lounge daily!) The despair in fact increased as the consequences on my career of a second serious suicide attempt sank in. That vicious circle of depression playing on the terrible state of my life, leading to a deepening of the depression and so on... was causing a downward spiral that was worse than what I had endured before my latest cry for help. In fact, the suicide attempt was assuredly a symptom of treatment failure *despite* being in hospital for almost *six months!*

CANCER REARS ITS UGLY HEAD

My idea of complications was just about to take almost an almost fiction novel-like turn. One day not long after being released from the ICU, I was lying in bed and experienced sudden onset of severe shortness of breath. Despite having my roommate tell my nurse about this, no one came for about half an hour. When she did come, the nurse tried to tell me to calm down as it was only "a panic attack". About the only time that I pushed my status as a physician, I demanded that a non-invasive measurement of my oxygen levels be done. This involves a clip being placed on the finger, which gives one an instantaneous measure of pulse rate and oxygen saturation in blood. Normal for oxygen is anything above 92 per cent. My values were in the *low eighties.*

After noting this, the nurse became upset having no "medical" training as such. My psychiatrist was called and an urgent consult was made to an Internal Medicine specialist. I was left on oxygen and the specialist arrived within thirty minutes. I underwent some special tests and was shown to have bilateral, multiple pulmonary emboli (numerous blood clots in both lungs). These arise most often from prolonged immobilization (plane/car trips, but in this case I later found out that during my hospital stay in my home town after the suicide attempt, I had *not been placed* on blood thinner injections that prevent these type of clots!) In a terrible case of irony, I had at one time been involved in worldwide published research on the effect of cancer on the increased risk of pulmonary emboli.

I was quickly transferred to a medical ward and started on urgent blood thinner by intravenous, later to be replaced by daily injections for a year. A *hospitalist* (again irony raised its ugly head, the position that I founded in this hospital over ten years previously, and the first full-time program of its type in the country) examined me for admission to the floor. It was the first thorough medical exam I had received out of all the encounters I had received (first and second suicide attempts, stays in ICU, admission to psychiatry ward twice). She found a large mass on the side of my neck near the windpipe. In total honesty I had noticed this myself over months before my "fall from grace", but in a typical physician fashion ignored it, electing to take care of my patients first.

To summarize, several tests were done, including one of the most painful experiences I have ever experienced (including breaking bones, hockey injuries, major dislocation of my thumb, etc.) a needle biopsy of the thyroid. I knew, and almost expected now, the worst possibility in every turn of my life, and I was not disappointed. The biopsies and tests were positive for *metastatic thyroid papillary carcinoma*, in other words a very curable cancer of the thyroid that had spread to some local lymph nodes in the neck. (That's why showering in the filthy showers mentioned earlier had actually been *dangerous* to my immune-compromised state with cancer!)

Normally, a surgery would have been done followed by radiation, but the new blood thinner situation and lung clots complicated things a lot. A period of treatment of my lungs was scheduled in which time the surgery/radiation would be postponed. Luckily the tumour was very slow growing and after surgery and radiation 95 per cent of patients with this cancer are free of disease at twenty years. Honestly, with the depression, fresh attempt at taking my life/ICU stay, lung clots and now cancer in less than a month, I was numb to anything going on, however had a very clear mind to appreciate the seriousness, if that makes any sense (see mention above of my research indicating higher risk of lung clots with my now diagnosed cancer).

Within a week or so I was returned to the *dungeon.* A new consciousness about my health was expressed by the nurses and doctors, half because I feel they had self-realization of their negligence, and half not to be caught off guard again.

IT WASN'T ALL TERRIBLE

A few of my bright spots were three families from my practice who somehow found out where *I lived now* and visited me in hospital over fifteen months (outside of lawyers, bankers; none of the twenty to thirty physicians in-house who I had worked with for five years ever visited or said hi, even when one who had been a next door neighbour visited his daughter admitted to the psychiatry unit) and the ongoing support of my father. Because of the circumstances, I never had outside privileges or my own clothes for a long time. About two months after my lung and cancer diagnoses, some minor drug changes were made but again had little effect on the depression even after months.

A constant positive in my life, also present during my hospitalization, is a friendship of almost 40 years with R.

She and I met in our early teens when we were in Air Cadets in my hometown in Atlantic Canada. We were part of a very close knit group of friends, both male and female, who did almost everything together. Although there has never been anything romantic between R. and me, over the years as other friendships fell by the wayside, ours remained strong. We helped each other through relationship problems and break ups, the very difficult births of her two boys, deaths in the family and whatever else that life brought our way. However we always have had a good laugh together, making fun of one another, recalling the past and enjoying the newest additions to her family, her two grand babies!

Even when I have been distracted by work or other stressors, R. has always been there. At times when I have neglected to call back, she remains persistent and eventually with some smart aleck remark on my voicemail gets me to call!

Most importantly, she has remained in my corner through the recovery that I have had to make from the events that I have yet to finish describing.

On two or three occasions I found gross blood in my urine while on blood thinners. My nurse on each occasion was shown the blood in the toilet. A "urine sample" was taken and nothing further was done or said by a physician. In fact this should have been an indication for a full urologic work up and stoppage of the anti-coagulation therapy if warranted.

Nothing was done.

About three months after diagnosis, my time for surgery arrived. It involved being transferred across the city to another hospital. It was a bitter cold winter causing people to "be depressed". I was finally speaking with my father, especially since the lung clot and cancer diagnosis. Despite having been there for my mom for about fifty years with her depression, he still scolded me for the suicide attempts saying, "But you're a doctor!" (a phrase I have heard innumerable times since and even today *much* to my chagrin). It was as if to say the Hippocratic Oath has some protective power over all sworn to its content. In fact, at least 50 per cent of physicians have a substance dependence disorder and/or mental health diagnosis. The actual reported incidence is much smaller, as doctors do not reveal their issues *exactly* because of what has happened to me subsequent to my revelation!

Another kick in the teeth was that none of my family was traveling to be with me for my surgery. In fact, my father and brother were booked for a two-week holiday to visit relatives in California exactly over the time of my surgery and post-operative recovery. They argued that they really could not do anything but sit with me while *I wouldn't talk to them anyway and that the trip had been booked for such a long time.* There was some truth to this, but to have someone there for a serious operation would have been nice.

The operation went well as I was told, but I had to stay at this hospital until my drains stopped putting out blood. I had a semi-private room, with no one bugging me and my own personal TV swivelling into my bed. I literally prayed each day that my stay would have to be prolonged. I actually stayed a bit longer due to my drain. But, it finally was time to return to the psychiatric ward. My healing went on very well. Usually the systemic radiation (treatment given internally as pill to cover the entire body) was given two to three months after surgery but this was again complicated by my blood thinning treatment for my lung clots and delayed.

Another problem was associated with the radiation. After swallowing the radioactive capsule, one must stay in an isolated lead-lined room for up to five days while the radioactivity becomes less dangerous in your body fluids. The radiation specialists were concerned that I might harm myself while in isolation treatment. Even in my depressed state, I wanted to rid my body of the cancer and additional waiting for radiation added yet another unbelievable layer to my worry and non-healing mood. The radiation was delayed for almost two to three months beyond normal treatment times due to the *negotiations ongoing between the psychiatrists and nuclear medicine doctors.*

At no time was I asked for an opinion.

In the interim, a loony plan was hatched that I was ready for discharge. I was no better than the day I had been admitted and an argument can be made that I was worse with all the life-altering medical news I had endured of late. The problem was that despite the state of my health, I wanted *out*, due to the dismal atmosphere of the ward and my very real opinion as both a doctor and patient (admittedly a complicated relationship) that nothing was being done for me in hospital.

The other major issue was that I had nowhere to go. My social worker was absolutely useless in this regard and discharge planning is almost solely a primary task of SW especially with psychiatric patients. Luckily another social worker took over in his vacation absence and she was wonderful at that time and later on when I would be finally discharged. My estranged wife had sold the house and lived with a sister for a while (until mysteriously she moved within ten kilometres of me *after* I was discharged from hospital). I therefore had no close friends with whom I could stay who understood my complicated circumstance. The psychiatrist had no helpful suggestions either, so once again I was left to my devices to fend for myself in a severely depressed state. My protestations that I was not ready for discharge fell on deaf years.

As I have mentioned, a few friends and patients did visit me in hospital. One of these set of friends were the mother and father of a high school student I had hired part-time in my office, and as luck would have it at the same time the brother and sister-in-law of a full-time employee.

They graciously offered their home as a *temporary* launching point from which to start a new life for myself. As much as I was unsure of the discharge I was elated to escape from "emotional Alcatraz". I was discharged with just three grocery bags of belongings.

Another complication is that my estranged wife wanted all my possessions removed from the home since possession by the new owners was imminent. She unilaterally moved my belongings into a storage depot with no respect for equal division of property, choosing the newer and better of everything. I arrived with my sport utility vehicle – SUV – recently given to me by my partner because of her claim that she couldn't pay for it and with my high school employee (now co-hostess at my new digs) as a witness. We had one hour to remove everything that had not been packed by movers. Even with my friend's help it took over an hour with the SUV packed to the point of being almost unsafe for visibility.

The possessions and SUV were left in the back of the driveway of my new temporary lodgings with hopes that I would be moving into my own place within weeks. It is important to remember that over a half year of being on an anti-depressant, it was *abruptly stopped* and not continued as a discharge medication. This is widely known to cause a potentially *very dangerous* syndrome called Antidepressant Discontinuation Syndrome, which I did go on to suffer due to the psychiatrist's negligence.

The signs were on the wall. On only a mood stabilizer without an anti-depressant, I was bound to sink deeper into a depression. No follow-up post-discharge was planned for one month.

Things began favourably. I honestly wanted to get outside and do chores, vacuum, walk the dog twice daily and help as I could around the house. The lady of the house would leave town up to four to five days to take care of her grandchildren and I would even cook for her husband and myself in her absence, though this simple chore would cause great anxiety.

Insidiously my interest in everything slowed, almost imperceptibly over weeks. We played scrabble as a "family" all at the mercy of the man of the house who was undisputed champion. We laughed a lot, and even though I was perennially third or fourth out of four, I truly enjoyed our game nights usually coincident with dessert and coffee. But soon this was a chore (anhedonia the big medical word, again) as well.

By the sixth week the lady of the house, rightfully so, reminded me occasionally about our promise of this being my *temporary* step to recovery. However as time went on I retrogressed and by the end, was staying in bed twenty-four hours a day huddled in a state of now "underground" depression. (Not a surprise from the medication omission I mentioned earlier!).

ANOTHER SUICIDE ATTEMPT

One night in *yet another* fit of desperation, I lied to my male host and said that I was going to dinner at a friend's house. At this point I still had a key to my office amazingly, with *all* the previous goings on. I sat in the office for hours deliberating the recent and past events and what action I could carry out in response to the dismal situation and long term hopelessness. Again in the throes of an *untreated bipolar type II* depression, ending my life was the answer. I left the house at 6:00 p.m. Until 2:00 a.m. I slowly dosed myself with blood pressure pills to the point I was so hypotensive that I couldn't get up from a chair. My blood pressure was so low that I couldn't do it on the office machine because I couldn't get up and see the numbers clearly. These symptoms stayed with me for two or three days, more or less. As a result of the overdose, my kidney function deteriorated severely and was never even noted by my psychiatrist until I pointed it out. (It was only upon my insistence that this was addressed by a kidney specialist!)

By the grace of God only, I drove home that night safely unable to see straight. My only regret was the consternation I caused my male host. He stayed up until 3:00 a.m. God Bless him, worrying about me. He had even wanted to call the police but I had called him in the intervening period thankfully. I made my apologies very curtly and collapsed into bed for the next few days.

The breaking point was when I did not attend my psychiatric follow-up appointments and erased the messages from voicemails so that my hosts would not find out about my delinquency. One day the psychiatrist contacted my hostess directly and the jig was up. In her defence, my friend and hostess was one for tough love. To this day I remember the enforced grilled cheese sandwich and tea she made me eat and drink on the back patio after a much-needed shower and a shave. She informed me that the psychiatrist wanted her to bring me in for admission the next day, but before that she wanted the entire contents of the SUV emptied into the basement so that my ex could pick up the vehicle, which was blocking the end of her driveway. For a person with not enough energy to get out of bed, I single-handedly moved the entire contents of the vehicle, with my hostess and daughter packing it in their already crowded basement. To this day I have no idea what became of those boxes.

The next fateful day as I counted off the minutes overnight, my hostess drove me to the hospital and gave me a genuine hug for recovery, but left me at the steps of Hades nonetheless. My welcome to the psychiatric ward was awkward due to the unsuccessful discharge only weeks ago or due to simple indifference.

A very important note is that each time I was readmitted it was through the ER. At no point did an ER physician touch me for an exam and no blood work done after a known *"repeat overdose patient"* was readmitted to psychiatry with an admission of longer than six months.

In reality it was as is if I had never left. The nurses, doctors and staff's attitude had not changed. It was as if their world had stood still but mine had sunk even further despite their ignorance.

I stayed off anti-depressant for months. The situation went from bad to worse. Things had not changed for me despite a suicide attempt out of hospital, a premature discharge, second suicide attempt, cancer diagnosis and surgery, recalcitrant depression over six months in hospital and occult third suicide attempt with acute kidney failure.

Amazing...

At this point in my life I was on autopilot with no real concept of life's ups and downs, as all that I had experienced of late were downs. Patients that were friends on the ward became annoyances, I was slightly more verbal about treatment recommendations by non-physician staff and I was slowly losing all my confidence in my psychiatrist.

JUST WHEN I THOUGHT THINGS COULDN'T GET ANY WORSE THEY DID!

One day as I was in bed I had sudden onset of severe right abdominal pain. Again, having been used to several types of pain, I put up with it until about an hour from onset. The nurses only half believing in its existence gave me acetaminophen. The medication may well have been water as thirty minutes later the pain had worsened.

The nurses had only orders for repeating the acetaminophen, which might have been a placebo in regards to its efficacy, but that is all they offered. They refused to contact the MRP despite my pleas. Ironically, they should have known that I would not cry wolf with all that I had been through. Regardless, the pain went on for a total of eight hours from its onset when they finally received an order for a paltry dose of acetaminophen with codeine from the psychiatrist, who knows little or nothing about abdominal pain.

The pain was so severe that I could not sit or lie and did countless rounds of the ward staring at the nurses who seemingly were ignoring my pain. Finally after *twelve hours* since onset of the pain, and no relief whatsoever, a surgeon was called. An hour later a student working with the surgeon (resident) came to the floor. She examined me and verified what I had thought all along that I was suffering from a gallbladder attack. The surgeon was in the OR and gave consent to administer a very strong pain medication. *Sixteen hours* after the onset of my pain, I finally had relief.

Two hours later, the surgeon came down, ordered an urgent CT scan of my abdomen which showed a gangrenous (infected, rotting) gallbladder. I was too sick to have an operation and was transferred to the surgical ward for continuous pain medication and high dose intravenous antibiotics for days. It would take three weeks for me to be well enough to have an operation.

As 'luck' would have it this fell into a fortuitous timeframe. Remember that my radiation specialists had trepidation about doing a four to five day treatment behind closed doors. They reasoned that if I survived surgery admission I could be trusted with my post-surgical cancer treatment.

RADIATION: A TRULY WELCOME RESPITE!

The fact that I looked forward to being locked in a room by myself for five days should be a statement yet again of my state of mind and mood. I survived radiation without problems after being in radiation lock-up. I did have some tongue sores and painful, swollen salivary glands post-radiation, but these are well known side effects of this particular type of treatment. It was heaven, with my own TV and computer access in over a year and solitary peace. I returned to the psychiatry ward when I was no longer radioactive. Within a few weeks of my recovery I had my gallbladder surgery and returned to the ward the day after the operation.

I was given a single room for a few days out of courtesy for all my medical ailments. My blood thinning for my lung clots had to be also very carefully considered.

Probably a month after my cancer radiation and gallbladder surgery I was considered to be well again from a medical perspective. Little did I know I know that I had received treatment without my consent!

A new vogue in depression is use of a drug called ketamine. It amazingly is a conscious sedation drug, that is to say it is most often used in the ER when someone has to be 'put under' but still breathing on their own while having a painful procedure (broken bone set, child needing many stitches, etc.). It is also used when wanting to intubate a person (put breathing tube in) or even deliver an electric shock to the heart while a person is awake. In many of these cases it is also used in conjunction with a potent painkiller.

However, its first use was and still is in the OR where it is used with other anaesthetic agents for general anaesthesia. I am unsure of how the utility for depression was discovered, but I assume that someone with depression underwent a conscious sedation or general anaesthesia and awoke sometime later with an improvement in their depression. It is now given by infusion intermittently, that is intravenously over some period of time and then at intervals as dictated by the response to the drug.[10] (Recently a huge controversy has arisen in the United States where ketamine has been used alone or with other drugs for lethal injection capital punishment. There is no standardization of the doses and some events have resulted in so-called "botched" executions where inmates have died in agonizing ways with incorrect use of ketamine.)

Unbeknownst to me, my psychiatrist asked the anaesthetist on my gallbladder case to add ketamine to my anaesthesia. The results were possibly beneficial, but broke a basic tenant of medicine – consent to treatment of which I was totally capable at the time. I suppose the thought was a "depressed" psychiatric patient had no right to consent. *I did not learn of the use of the ketamine until after three years post-discharge from hospital.*

Despite the ketamine, I did not feel better up to one to two months after my operation. *I* had to request that my psychiatrist add an anti-depressant (the fear at times of these drugs that even with a mood stabilizer, the addition can bring on mania or hypomania).

THE ADMINISTRATION DECIDED I SHOULD BE DISCHARGED!

As per the subtitle above, my psychiatrist readily agreed; I would soon learn why. By this time I had been in hospital about fourteen months. The *administration* of the hospital decided I had been in hospital long enough. According to the psychiatrist he had no say in the matter. SW (the helpful female one) did recognize that I was incapable of living independently, so they sent me on a tour of two senior citizens' "resorts" despite my protests that I didn't feel secure being discharged. The anti-depressants had still not started to take effect and a profound anxiety set in, understandable for someone who had been in hospital for that long and with my diagnosis.

It was about a month before discharge and as usual no one was listening to my accounting of what *my* needs were. Disposition after a crazy admission of fifteen months (agreed upon by *all* my physicians) was being decided by non-medical people. The source of these decisions with seemingly no say by my psychiatrist made me even more insecure. The nurses were made aware that I didn't think I was ready to go, the psychiatrist really didn't care and I was left to stew in this dangerous mixture of depression, lack of confidence and energy-sapping anxiety. Time seemed to be flying towards my release from a place that I once would have paid a million dollars to exit. The parties *deciding my exodus obviously had no knowledge of my clinical history and likely didn't care.*

Once again I was given no other choice but to adopt my own treatment plan as suboptimal as it may have been. I again absconded from the hospital on a pass to go walking. I got a bus to a walk-in clinic and innocently requested a thirty day supply of blood pressure pills, plus bought an antiemetic (against nausea) and antihistamine to put me asleep. I think that on the basis of my personal history, you can predict what came next.

ANOTHER CRY FOR HELP

I chose a small inconspicuous motel in the periphery of town and took all the pills that I could without vomiting. I had had nothing to eat or drink for thirty-six hours and had prepaid in cash for three days, thinking the event would be all over by then. I did nothing but sleep. I think it was little after the thirty-six hour mark that a harsh knocking woke me from what I had hoped was going to be *my terminal slumber*. I stumbled to the door and found a big policeman and petite policewoman waking me from my drug-induced stupor. I verified my identity and they instructed me that they were there to bring me back to the hospital. They were very understanding, much more so than the reception I anticipated that would await me upon my return to the hospital.

Again I was first was seen in the ER where not a drop of blood was drawn on an overdose patient, and the *doctor's exam* consisted of a cursory, "Are you OK?" without any touch.[III]

Incredibly, on not one of the screenings post-overdose was any sort of physical examination done, blood work for other drugs (something that is "Standard of Practice") or neurologic evaluation performed. I don't know if this was again because of the fact that I was a psychiatric patient, but in my personal experience as an ER doc, it was tantamount to malpractice.

An interesting sidebar is that several years after I left hospital, I recounted to a prominent lawyer the *numerous* malpractices that I had suffered. Considering the multiple episodes of negligence I had endured, I asked about possible litigation. His actual advice to a now very well physician was, *"As a bipolar patient you will never be able to win a malpractice suit because they will bring up your mental health as an argument."*

That is where the judicial system sits for wrongdoings against mental health patients. I hope that another book will address the unending litany of these human rights breaches by government, the Department of National Defence, the legal system, business and society. The stigma of falsehoods associated with psychiatric patients involving all these bodies would also be addressed. I referred to a revolving door admission pattern with psychiatric patients with data supported from studies. These patients were at least discharged for some time. I seemed to be readmitted within the same admission! This made me either *special,* or as I think, resulted from *medical and psychiatric malpractice.*

My psychiatrist seemed to be a lot more sympathetic with this suicidal attempt, saying, "I was up all night calling the hospital every two hours about you!" My feeling was that now I had attempted suicide four times "on his watch", as we said in the military, it was

---

III   I know the name of the physician to this day and remember his disinterested face.

only a matter of time before the College of Physicians and Surgeons in our jurisdiction might respond to such a dismal record with severe sanctions. Despite the aforementioned legal opinion, I still today in the clear light of time still consider litigation.[IV]

Years after leaving hospital I ran across this investigative piece by the internationally renowned W5 documentary investigative team from CTV in Canada.[11] The piece hit home in a thunderclap fashion as I had almost successfully committed suicide while under psychiatric care *four* times (once when I should never have been discharged), along with a lifetime stain on my professional and personal reputation due to premature discharge on another occasion. Can one be safe in the place everyone sends you when you are in the greatest risk of self-harm? Where else is there to go?

I was once more settled in to my "home for now" but amazingly the reason for my latest suicide attempt was ignored despite my *recurrent* anxieties about discharge from hospital, suboptimal depression treatment and general deconditioning from society. Nevertheless, the counter ticked for my date to leave hospital like the timer rolling down to a bomb exploding. The anti-depressant that *I* had suggested weeks earlier was kicking in. A faint ray of hope seemed to be emerging. The problems facing me upon discharge were profound however: finances, professional, permanent residence, destroyed reputation, just to name a few. As I became more acclimatized to the idea of leaving hospital forever, things that I had hidden at the back of my mind to deal with came to the fore. At this point I was so devoid of

---

IV   This same psychiatrist was the MRP of a physician (in the hospital where I was the first hospitalist) who had an in-hospital *liaison* with an operating room nurse that went bad. After the doctor was spurned (under the care of the psychiatrist) he stalked the target of his affections and one night when they were alone in the hospital shot her fatally. Shortly thereafter he committed suicide by shooting himself in a nearby park. A huge provincial inquiry/coroner's case ensued which has resulted in permanent protective-security measures in that hospital and more far flung. My psychiatrist had to testify at the hearings and I am unsure whether he was reprimanded.

resolve that I developed the attitude that things would have to take care of themselves.

PEOPLE WITH MENTAL HEALTH ISSUES HAVE PRIDE

I was forced to decide on a seniors' retirement home on the basis of what I could afford. It was clean and otherwise pleasant, but the idea of mine having had a thriving medical practice less than a year and a half ago, and now having to live somewhere I would have placed a patient, was not only disheartening but a blow to my pride. Even people with mental health illnesses have pride.

    D-day finally arrived and with four shopping bags now containing my life's belongings I went by taxi to the seniors' home. My estranged wife had a vehicle but refused to give it to me. I was relegated to taxis for the next three months or walking to places near to the residence. The residents – all at least thirty or forty years older than me – were for the most part a welcome change of compassion and some even parental surrogates. Over the six months I lived there I felt welcome but at the same time a foreigner in a land of people living to survive to the end, while I was trying to survive to live to another beginning.

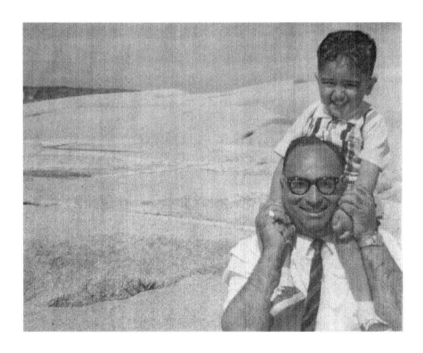

Picture of me and my Dad, my age 30 months old, 1966.

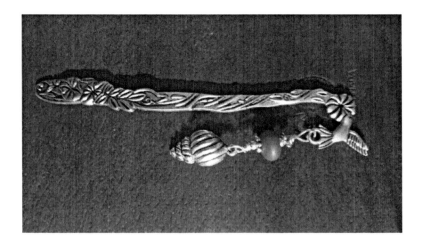

Bookmark given to me by a housekeeper from my hospitalization of 15 months from 2010-2011.

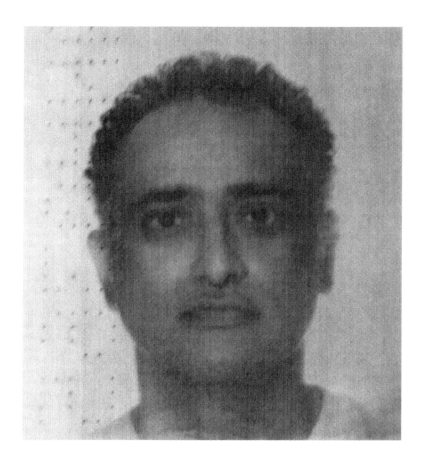

Picture of me 1 month post discharge from hospitalization of 15 months, August 2011.

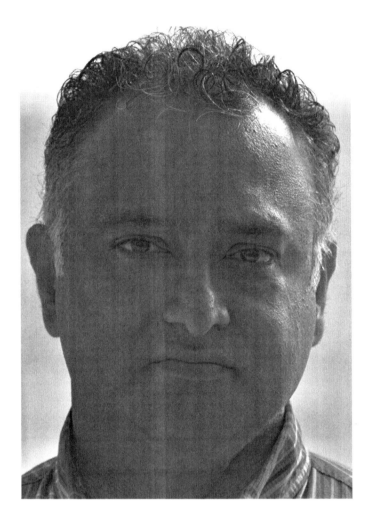

Picture of me 3 years post discharge from hospital in Mexico, January 2015.

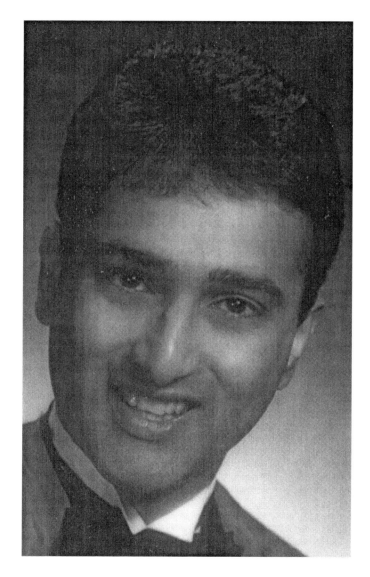

Medical school graduation picture 1990.

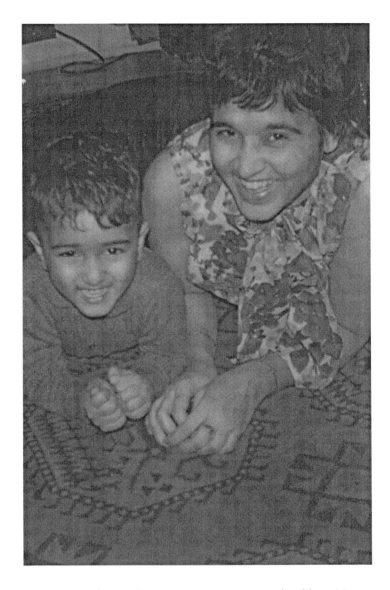

Picture of me and my Mom, my age 30 months old, 1966.

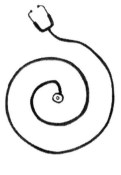

Chapter 3

THE BATTLE TO HAPPINESS

Very soon I had to come to grips with the issues that I had been lamenting before I left hospital. To sum it up – I had lost everything.

1.

The first issue was my estranged wife. Through some lawyer friends I retained one of the best divorce attorneys in the province. The complainant (as my wife will be known from now on) hired a much lesser lawyer. From the beginning the demands were totally out of the realm of legal reality. For example she demanded a personal care allowance of $10,000 per month, knowing that my disability allowance was a fraction of her demands. My counsel was an extremely wise and patient lawyer and we went through a two year battle of the complainant making ridiculous demands but not answering for six months after our response. She kept a small vehicle despite the fact that I was paying the monthly payments. The luxury vehicles were all returned. Within three months of being at the seniors' residence my lawyer demanded, rightfully for several medical reasons, that I required the vehicle. After a month's wait I did get the car so I was able to get around the city more easily, which is quite spread out.

Eventually after two years the divorce was finally signed with *some* financial issues still open, which I left totally to my counsel. Unfortunately, the complainant continues to this day to make my life difficult in any imaginative way she can. My counsel has become so tired of the affair that he does my work pro bono. The unending barrage of ludicrous annoyances no longer bothers me. Life over the time I have described to you has taught me in an oft-used adage: Do not to sweat the small stuff! *Really!*

2.

The second problem was that upon getting access to the Internet, I saw there were many newspapers local and out of town that had written totally one-sided articles about me from the now settled legal case, to me having abandoned my patients. <u>No follow-up articles treated the side of the story where all charges had been dropped and the complainant discredited by both the police and the College of Physicians and Surgeons</u> which handles all complaints against doctors; especially treating any suspected sexual impropriety by doctors extremely harshly. Even after the above judgements in my favour, the media articles on Google persisted. I tried every method offered by Google to remove the clearly libellous charges, even writing to the newspapers involved directly. My private medical life was available to the entire Internet to see! Appendix 3. To date, some of the articles have disappeared but Appendix 3 shows the height of the disastrous effects to my reputation.

Luckily, Google is now having to deal with European complaints of third party web postings harmful to one's reputation. I only hope it comes to North America soon. Again refer to Appendix 3 for my web solution to begin "damage control".

The best friends growing up who never have called since those fifteen months, family friends, medical colleagues and even non-medical associates, persist until today, due to the stigma of dealing with a mental health patient. Not Rohit, the person. Over 30-50 per cent of physicians likely have mental health and/or substance abuse disorder (of this latter group 90 per cent have a mental health diagnosis).

No wonder getting a *doctor* to a *doctor* for care or admitting that they need one is difficult, let alone convincing a doctor to do a study on fellow doctors, and press the panic button in society!

Read on.

What is truly astounding is that a careful search of the literature found only one study pointing to definite statistics on mental health disease among physicians: "The prevalence of common mental disorders among hospital physicians and their association with self-reported work ability: a cross-sectional study."

—BMC Health Serv Res. 2012 Aug 31;12:292-8

3.

As I have mentioned, the only reason that I lost my licence to practice medicine is that my ex-wife did not bring me the annual renewal forms. In fact, had I renewed the licence and gone through everything that I had in the fifteen months, my licence would likely have been held temporarily until I had recovered from my illness. The College in our province was so adamant about this anomaly in regulations regarding licence renewal, that pleas on the part of my psychiatrist, the Canadian Medical Protection Association (CMPA)[V] lawyer, cancer doctors, family doctor, nationally-renowned

---

V CMPA is the body that defends doctors in complaints or legal claims brought against them and most other advice concerning the legalities of the practice of medicine.

sub-specialty psychiatrists and the Physician Help Program (PHP) fell on deaf ears.[VI]

My reapplication was very suspicious regarding the CPSO response from the very beginning in that it took over a year and a half to be considered (usually about six months). It was supported wholeheartedly by the PHP along with my psychiatrist. Over that time I appeared before several committees of the College who questioned me about:

> 1) My mental health (cleared by PHP and my psychiatrist)
>
> 2) Previous patient complaints by patients – likely during periods when I was not treated properly for my bipolar disorder (these complaints came from only ONE place that I had worked at in all my career; racially motivated I feel, corroborated by several visible minority physicians who had worked in that area and left for that reason!). No further action on any of these complaints went to the Discipline Committee of the CPSO, where all serious matters regarding physician conduct are sent.
>
> 3) Ability to practice medicine (was awarded *Letter of Commendation from Registrar of College of Physicians and Surgeons of Ontario on asset to medical profession and bringing the art to practice of medicine 1998*) with no committee evidence brought up about any misgivings about same.

[VI] PHP is a part of our provincial medical association (our "union" so to speak) that treats and monitors doctors with mental health and substance dependence issues.

4) The sexual assault allegation against me that was found to be groundless (although splattered in the media with no retraction after all charges had been dropped!).

In the end, all the committees refused to make a decision either for or against my application. At each stage of the process my decision date with the Registration Committee was postponed further.

Finally a refusal of my application was decided, again with *no stated reason* that is customary under such circumstances.

In discussions with several other doctors, my family doctor, a nationally-renowned psychiatrist who reviewed my case, multiple physician therapists who saw me, the CMPA (not in so many words as to stay politically correct), a prestigious law firm in Toronto with one of the top specialized lawyers in the province for health law and even the PHP and my psychiatrist, all believed that "Something was rotten in the state of Denmark!"

In yet another twist of fate, my psychiatrist of eleven years after having written letters to the College saying that, "Dr. Kumar's *non-return to work* would be injurious to his health," suddenly was not supportive of same. In an equally bizarre occurrence, the PHP, which had overwhelmingly supported my return to the practice of medicine also agreed with the psychiatrist (not entirely surprising as they usually have to go by what the MRP says).

There had been no recurrence of symptoms, concerns by people watching me (my common-law partner at the time, close friends, my family doctor) or increases in medication. In fact there were dose decreases that I did not really want to take!

As previously mentioned, I think that my psychiatrist felt that he had been burned in the other physician case under his care with the disastrous outcome of a homicide/suicide. It can only have coloured his opinion. It certainly would have mine in his position, however this is not the way medicine should be practiced.

This now almost two year battle to return to my vocation and life's passion did break me temporarily I must admit.

I even appealed to the CMPA to help, but even a letter to the president of that body was refused despite my extenuating circumstances. Their policy was not to get involved with registration issues. Several levels at the CMPA including the president wished me "good luck with your future."

I hired the law firm and counsel discussed above and have spent up to $50,000 to reapply to the College. We are currently in a reevaluation phase. My longstanding psychiatrist and I mutually parted ways after what I thought were illogical decisions about my future, based on no sound clinical reason. I now have a much better psychiatrist who sees me as a whole person, not as one with a somewhat tragic recent history who should be protected from himself and the practice of medicine in an extremely paternalistic manner. This latter form of practice by any physician is highly frowned upon.

5.

A very real problem that I encountered upon leaving my sheltered twenty-one months was that my formerly very comfortable financial status built up over twenty-five years was shattered!

Due to negligence on the part of my ex-wife, credit cards had remained unpaid, personal and corporation taxes were neglected to a tune of $200,000 combined (not *her* personal taxes) and my office building remained unsold. All my personal and business credit cards had a balance of over $20,000, though she too was a co-signatory on these cards.

Despite the fact that I paid off all the credit cards at one time and had several physicians attest to the extenuating circumstances, all my cards were canceled. These cards were needed to launch my reapplication for a medical licence and generally get me back on my feet. I eventually got a credit card through some connections at a bank. It until today remains my only credit card.

A business line of credit also co-signed by my ex-wife of $40,000 outstanding debt continues to be paid by me to this day as well.

Luckily, in a case of divine intervention, I met up with a bankruptcy trustee who was able to negotiate my $200,000 tax debt to $60,000. To this day I remain very close to this person who now is more of a spiritual guide and mother figure in my life. My new accountant has also been a Godsend in my life, organizing the chaos of corruption, deceit and mismanagement of which I have been a victim.

My office building remained on the market for two years, low on the priority of the realtors. In yet another cruel turn in my rather unfortunate fate, one of the realtors was the spouse of the malpracticing accountant who may have aided my ex-wife in her embezzlement. The building has since been sold at a loss.

6.

Aftercare, which is the make-or-break criteria for many illnesses such as substance dependence, cancer care and mental health care is largely non-existent in our country. This issue along with compliance is the reason for what we call revolving door admissions to psychiatric wards. Worldwide research shows that these admissions account for up to 40 per cent of patients in a psychiatric ward at any time, and represent the highest prevalence of patients.

As you will see later, this huge cost to our economy is an indicator that there is a *systemic* breakdown in the way mental health patients are treated. Almost nowhere else in health care do you see this amount of repetition in hospital readmission. It has to be noted however for fairness, that I have already pointed to non-compliance on the part of patients as a partial contributor to this problem. However, if more time was spent with patients, educating them about side effects, the importance of compliance and overall resulting quality of life, this would be less of a problem. (Over fifteen years I timed outpatient psychiatric visits between three and five minutes in various psychiatrists' offices!)

In all frankness and fairness again, psychiatric patients have a tendency to also be not so innocent in the overall breakdown of our system. Some are extremely manipulative, at times due to their diagnoses such as personality disorders, or as a result of the stigma and dismissal by aftercare, forcing them to be "resourceful" in getting attention or resources. A great example is the **only** way mental health patients can enter the health care system at present throughout our country.

REPEATERS USE THE "S" WORD FOR INSTANT ADMISSION

There is no such thing as an elective referral to a psychiatrist in our country, that is if a family doctor wants a mental health patient referred to a psychiatrist, the delay can be six months to greater than a year depending on the jurisdiction. That means that a potentially ill patient must wait for care. The out is always, "If they are that sick then send them to the ER." In order for a patient to be seen by a crisis worker (usually a specialized RN or student doing a psychiatry rotation *not* a psychiatrist) the patient must be a harm to themselves or others. Repeaters have therefore learned that the "S" word (suicidal ideation not attempt) is *a get into jail free card* and direct admission ticket usually, as long as there are enough beds. Most times there are not, and patchwork remedies must be arranged. Patients who do not have family doctors do arrive in true crisis such as post-suicide attempts – conscious or unconscious arrest by police, domestic abuse, mental illness masking as substance dependence, motor vehicle accidents caused by mental diagnoses, etc. They usually also very often get treated for the "face" diagnosis and the mental health diagnosis goes by.

If one looks at almost all mass, psychopathic or *weird* murders (non-domestic), there was always an early sign in childhood, adulthood *or* even an ignored cry for help by the murderer, and I maintain, victim as well. The most recent in our country were the senseless murders in October 2014 of a member of the Canadian Armed Forces standing guard at the National War Memorial and another Forces member in Quebec about the same time. After the killing of the assailants, it was discovered that they had several times sought psychiatric help in another province and had been refused or ignored.

Another gruesome incident was a stabbing murder, beheading and cannibalism in front of an entire Greyhound passenger complement in 2008. The perpetrator was judged clinically insane with severe schizophrenia. A first responder police officer committed suicide in July 2014 after a long struggle with PTSD from this incident. There were signs of deteriorating health in the murderer, not picked up by his wife or employees. He was a highly-trained computer scientist, now a Canadian citizen, trained in China and doing menial jobs since immigrating to Canada.

Yet another inquiry is ongoing at present of a police shooting of a "street person" in Montreal. Before he went to the streets he had two children and was a well-respected molecular biologist. He was found downtown Montreal swinging a hammer at police asking them to, "Go ahead and shoot me!" He had sought help twice for mental health concerns before going to the streets. He was shot fatally in cold blood.

Another tragic loss of a large number of innocent lives occurred when a Germanwings Airbus A320 jet plummeted into the French Alps in March 2015 as the co-pilot locked the pilot out of the cabin and purposefully crashed the jet in a suicide/mass murder gesture. Very quick investigation revealed failed psychiatric screening by the mother company, and giant in the industry, Lufthansa. Failure of the medical care system, the co-pilot's ex-girlfriend not reporting suspicious behaviour and threats to authorities and a series of checks and balances in the airline industry, caused a preventable tragedy, and hopefully a worldwide focus on this *universal* problem.

Even chronic pain (see magnitude of problem in a background letter I wrote in a subsequent chapter) is now known to have its roots in childhood trauma, that is, mental health issues. Our present techniques of dealing (or not dealing) with pain issues in the absence of dealing with emotional trauma, understandably results in the dismal success in treating chronic pain.

Lastly, as a former member of the Canadian Armed Forces and a military doctor with depression at the time, I was privy to the mishandling of mental health care in the Canadian military. As previously mentioned, a "suck it up" or "ignore it entirely" mentality abounded at the time.

AN EPIDEMIC OF SUICIDE IN THE CANADIAN ARMED FORCES

However, since then, combat and peacekeeping/combat missions in Somalia. Bosnia, Rwanda (high profile depression/PTSD case of Canadian UN force commander), Haiti and Afghanistan, have amplified this problem. A recent Auditor General report in December 2014 was very critical of the Canadian military's handling of mental health in general, not including the epidemic of PTSD-related suicides over the past several years. According to this report, 20 per cent of veterans wait greater than eight months for psychiatric help. The Canadian federal government in almost a pre-emptive move, announced days before this report that it would invest $200 million over six years on the psychiatric health care of Canadian soldiers. The reality of this announcement was that the announced money would actually be spent over 50 years not six as announced.

According to data from National Defence, 160 soldiers committed suicide between March 2004 and 2014 or more than were killed in combat in Afghanistan

—Toronto Star, Sept. 16, 2014

Another interesting and tragic study shows that in 2013, the Canadian Armed Forces had 2.5 times the number of suicides that the British forces did, even though it is only one-third the size. Obviously, Canadians are not doing or doing something very wrong compared to our British counterparts.

A national disgrace.

Another viewpoint is that of a recent editorial article in the Canadian Medical Association Journal (CMAJ), written by a medical doctor trained in Great Britain and the deputy editor of the CMAJ, commenting on the global and Canadian medical (mis)treatment of mental health patients. It's as though she read this book before she wrote the article.

An extremely tragic event involved a Japanese national in his forties who was beheaded by the notorious Islamic State of Iraq and Syria (ISIS) in January 2015.[12] Japanese officials knew of this victim as being, *"... An unstable man with a history of mental illness..."* as if family, friends, healthcare workers or the government could not have prevented his travel to an active war zone, especially in the age of universal fear of homegrown terrorism. What resulted was a horrific death of yet another mental health *victim,* in more than one sense of the word, for all the world to see in tragic real time.

The point is that these are the media-grabbing stories. Hundreds of thousands of Canadians have stories – perhaps not as dramatic – but equally destructive of their emotional lives, family, career and medical health. Too many end up in tragedy as I did as well.

I was lucky to escape my destruction, but still live with the consequences of the ineffective treatment of my disease every day.

Something has to give.

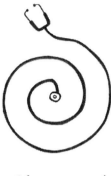

Chapter 4

BEWARE OF THE POWERS THAT BE...

The following letter, though somewhat cumbersome, is a letter to the leader of the federal Liberal party of Canada. A copy was also sent to the Dean of the local Law School and the Student Law Society (ostensibly/possibly some of our politicians of tomorrow) and also as an introduction and a reminder to a Department Head at the Ted Rogers School of Business MBA program who has agreed in principle with a collaboration, but as per the annotation below, has *not* acted on any discussion we have had to date.[VII]

In its circuitous route, it describes the aim of my corporation and my determination to write a law advocating for mental health

---

VII By the production phase of this book, the federal Liberal party leader, Dean of the Faculty of Law and Student Law society had *all* not had the decency of *even a reply*, to join the aforementioned addressees; a reinforcement of the apathy of today's leaders to these overwhelming mental health issues as pointed out in the letter and this book.

patients, substance dependence and chronic pain patients. It describes the horrible financial cost, and the human cost exemplified by my story, but is only one of hundreds of thousands of such stories across our nation.

Incredibly a member of the provincial parliament (MPP) was not interested in the bill, as was the case with a local economic and development corporation (headed by a former multiple cabinet minister at the provincial level, who was interestingly the CEO of a $1.54 billion annual revenue-generating juggernaut/utility monopoly, understandably not having time for my "disenfranchised" patients).

It remains to be seen if the Local Health Integration Network (LHIN) and a representative of the federal party in our riding may express interest.

Most notably however, a copy of the cover letter below was sent *to the CEO of the hospital where I had been admitted for fifteen months.* We had enjoyed some positive correspondence on favourable experiences, post-admission, I had had with non-psychiatric doctors at the institution and with loved ones of mine who attended the hospital as well. I received an appointment within days, but sent this cover letter with Mr. Trudeau's letter accompanying. The morning of the appointment I received a call from the CEO's secretary "that something has come up."

I have yet to hear back months thereafter! Not surprising I suppose for the head of the hospital where I had spent fifteen months of the worst days of my life!

Most recently I approached a prominent local producer/director at the local cable television station, after meeting her lovely daughter who was serving us at a local restaurant. The daughter is studying to be a part of the health care system and was interested in reading a rough draft of my book. I therefore wrote a very detailed email to her mother, the local cable executive, with a copy of my book for the daughter and a business proposal regarding promoting the cause of mental health in our community through local TV.

There has been no answer in over a month.[VIII]

Cover Letter (Email) to CEO

Hi _____,

Forgive the last minute agenda for my meeting with you tomorrow.

Below is a letter written to Justin Trudeau that gives some background on the general topic I want to address. The specifics arising from this summary for the purposes of our discussion are:

- The institution of a more intensive patient advocacy program at ___ expanding on the present program in place.
- The institution of above in the face of poor public perception of the ER at _____ campus as a single example only (too early discharge post-op in the eyes of patients, reputation of Surgical service, poor morale in Department of Family Medicine due to a certain staff member, public view of poor relations between members of Cardiology service, etc.)
- The collapsing palliative care program at _____campus (my sharing with an integral part of that program and our history together in co-implementation of one of the most successful new initiatives in ___ history; the Hospitalist Program). I authored one of the seminal papers in this country on the subject!

VIII The letter to Mr. Trudeau can be found at www.rtkumar.com

- Being one of the first hospitals in the nation to have such an advocacy program similar to the pioneering Hospitalist Program at _____ to which I contributed in a major fashion.
- Practical benefits of this proposal, most important of which would be improved bed utilization and shorter hospital stays with improved two-way communication with patient families and patients themselves.

All this in the multiple awards and recognitions I have received in my career regarding patient communication (see Awards and Distinctions section of C.V. - particularly proud of Commendation by the College of Physicians and Surgeons of Ontario.)

I trust that this provides us with ample fodder for a start for ongoing discussions, on a topic for which I have great passion. As with the offer to Mr. Trudeau, I could provide you with a rough draft only of my book (details about same in letter to Mr. Trudeau; unedited for copyright reasons) which may solidify for you the basis for my zeal!

I look forward to our meeting in person after so much correspondence!

Best regards,
Dr. Kumar (Tinni)

The struggle for mental health awareness affected me indirectly when I was about fifty years old, but illustrates this struggle clearly. I had always recognized in my medical practice that art therapy was beneficial for many mental health patients with some producing astonishing work. In fact a mainstay of treatment with many inpatient psychiatric units is to engage patients in daily occupational therapy, most of which is in multimedia artistic therapy. It is usually extremely well received by patients and staff alike.

To this end, in a medium sized city in southwestern Ontario where I was living at the time, the City Art, Cultural and Heritage department was sponsoring grants in an open competition with the stipulation that the main applicant must have a presence in the arts community locally. My brother-in-law at the time taught drawing at the local university along with animation. He was a well-respected animator in Hollywood having contributed to many major film projects with more than twenty years' experience in the industry at that level, indeed more than complying with the one stipulation of the grant process.

After the first round of funding we were unsuccessful, with reassurance that there had been a plethora of good candidates but choices had to be made and subsequently very good candidates including us were rejected. Having both experienced rejection in our professional life before, we took it all in stride.

For the second round of funding (both rounds were for $5000 CDN) I put in a lot of research background showing the aptitude of mental health patients in all types of artwork and the long established history of geniuses in all creative endeavours, many of whom had severe mental health disorders. We reasoned that such newfound works from an "unlikely" source would certainly enrich the art, culture and heritage of the community. To our surprise we did not get the $5000 funding, but the City in its inimitable wisdom chose to give $75,000 to summer students to clean the city's statues with toothbrushes all summer. Not only was this *15 times* the amount we requested, but five city workers who would require no extra funding, could have achieved the same with pressure hoses and some elbow grease within two days!

Your hard earned tax money at work folks *at the cost of a totally disenfranchised group in society!*

One result that I did expect from my illness but was still shocked to experience, was the total rejection by physicians who not only had been colleagues, but my family doctor, and even some who I had instructed in pain treatment and palliative care.

On one occasion I met one of these physicians at the grocery store. After some perfunctory comments she could not have made it more clear that she felt awkward and wanted "out of" the conversation and the meat aisle!

In another instance I was helping a friend with severe post-operative spinal surgery complications and pain. I had petitioned her family doctor years earlier for adequate analgesia with her history of longstanding, miraculous metastatic cancer survival. Despite the patient's constant pleas and complaints of drug side effects for three years, the family physician finally listened to me and put her patient on conservatively, *100 times* the amount of pain medication that she had been on, commenting, "Why didn't you tell me your pain was so bad?" after the fact in an admonishing manner, and voiced resentment towards me!

On this occasion post-operatively, in front of my ailing friend and her family, a family doctor who was one of my old colleagues (see AIDS doctor mentioned previously), *who I had taught* principles of pain management and now was the pain doctor on-call for pain treatment. He clearly ridiculed me in front of the patient when I asked a very pertinent question. What was worse, is that the son-in-law of the patient, a local specialist physician who had done nothing in the first three years of the patient's pain, now basically blocked me out of any contributions to her care, presumably partly out of embarrassment for his lack of participation, and partly due to my emotional turmoil to which he was privy. This occurred while the patient, who was totally competent, wanted me as part of her treatment team!

In another blow, several physicians who I had helped in the OR, to whom I had referred hundreds of patients, stabilized their patients in the ER, etc. for ten years, refused to give me references for my reapplication to obtain a licence to practice medicine. They all visited me in the ICU when I was self-harming, but now despite the written reassurances of my psychiatrist that *I should*, and was, capable to return to work, they rudely declined, not even responding to my written request.

It is no wonder that doctors do not want to reveal "frailties" of mental health illness and substance dependence, when the reaction from patients, colleagues, regulatory agencies and the public in general can be so polarized against them. Thank goodness in our province we do have the PHP for physicians. There are Employee Assistance Plans (EAPs) in the work force, but while in practice, I found that the support for mental health concerns was greatly behind that for substance abuse, as if the latter was better accepted in society, and likely is less stigmatized. Remember, 90 per cent of substance dependent individuals have mental health diagnoses.

"Frailties" are also something that families sometimes do not appreciate. My father is no exception.

After my discharge from hospital, our previously very close relationship was never the same. He actually warned me *not* to get into any other sexual harassment predicaments. He treated me as a patient, suggesting that I was not "capable" of work and should stay on the very comfortable tax-free disability until the age of sixty-five. When I returned home for four months getting a break from L. (our story to follow) he actually made me stay in a motel for two months while I was waiting for an apartment. He cited the fact that "my" personality was disruptive to him and my brother, who has always lived at home after finishing university never having worked in his life. I even made them dinner one night and dropped it off. They never reciprocated, other than an odd cup of tea, but even then hinted rather transparently when my stay was over.

They did let me "borrow" a pot and easy chair that had not been used for two decades, but just until my furniture arrived from my residence in another place in Canada.

I could not recall any one event that I may have perpetrated to deserve such treatment. All I know is that I was not welcome in a place that should have been a home.

Now my "baby" sister is an entirely different story...

DENIAL IS A DANGEROUS THING

Ever since my marriage to my second wife, relations went from great (the two of us taking care of her infant son overnight) to no contact. As far as I can recall there was a falling out between the two of them with no involvement with myself. Nevertheless, I no longer was able to see my soon-to-be two nephews. There was scant communication from her during all my life events, and even then indirectly through my father. We spoke once when my brother had a heart attack at age forty-five. Never was I contacted through the fifteen months in hospital or my ongoing stressors.

While I lived back home for the four months, I tried a reconciliation by email. It was met by a very non-committal "we'll see". The request was only to see my nephews who I had not seen in over eight to ten years. Although I had no definitive proof, I got the feeling that her reticence was on the basis of the fact that her brother was a sexual predator (though exonerated) and "a loony" that may go off on her boys at any time. This was just an excuse in the large scheme of things in my opinion.

I have tried to contact her since over the years and only received inexplicable verbal abuse, hostility and all out actions consistent with a personality disorder, one of the most difficult to treat psychiatric disorders. This is verified by written material I have retained and even feedback received from her workplace, very detrimental and almost contraindicated in her chosen profession. Look at the odds. With my mother and I both having significant, albeit in my case, now well-controlled mental health diagnoses, her odds of having a psychiatric disorder are greater than her risk of breast cancer (1:9 over her lifetime or 11 per cent) and risk of developing heart disease by the age of sixty-five, (28 per cent). The definition of a significant mental health diagnosis is one that affects your family life *or* occupation *or* physical health; only one needed. Two out of three fulfilled in my sister's case.

Through the media onslaught, "conspiracy" against my reapplication for a license, stigmatization by colleagues, friends, patients, family and society, loss of a marriage, financial ruin and having to rebuild a successful past that had taken forty-five years of *hard* work, you bet I felt discouraged and lacked the motivation to go on. But when I remembered patients through my career who faced much worse, children smiling with their bald little heads going through painful chemo, the faces of the majority of the world who struggle each day just to survive – *I felt rejuvenated to go on.*

A CONSIDERED WARNING

I consider myself to be a somewhat intelligent person not prone to be susceptible to "being taken". However, after discharge from hospital and very well-controlled from the perspective of my bipolar disorder, I was victim to two scams, one financial and one religious. People with mental health diagnoses are prone to both.

Dr. Andreasen, who I have quoted previously, points out that people with mental health disorders and creativity/intelligence (I humbly consider myself to have a bit of both) are more sensitive in a general way, sensitivity which also contributes to their talent as a creative brain.

In my case, I divulged my mental health history to a female in a business dealing and a male purporting to be a "Christian", in which a business dealing was also superimposed.

Big mistake. The first, an attractive female (see quote from Khalil Gibran later and studies regarding initial interaction between the sexes later in Chapter 5) who from the beginning "seemed" to share life views, ethics and views on business, not oft expressed by people in that field, for whom the bottom line is always the final word. She was different and we clicked from the beginning and later even in a 'romantic liaison of sorts'.

This person, saying all the right things, appealing to my sensitivity and sensibility, "took" me for $5000 CDN, not having contributed an iota to the promised work with my Corporation, which had been assured in a verbal and written contract. By the time I had consulted a dear friend who is a lawyer, she advised that it would be more expensive to recover the money than let it go. So I did.

This person knew of my mental history and I hers, severe co-dependence and father with issues of verbal abuse and abandonment. Her body habitus, BMI less than 15 suggested an eating disorder. Well-documented serial studies have shown that eating disorders are about greater than 90 per cent of the time associated with remote sexual abuse. She had enough on her plate to have me go through the negative energy *on my part* to litigate.

Religion is a solace that billions of people worldwide turn to in these troubled times that we deal with universally. Sometimes, patients with mental health disease lean on religion *(not faith)* more than non-affected people due to various reasons:

1. Desperation for belonging *to something* because society has rejected and stigmatized them.
2. Susceptibility to a message of hope that does not seem possible in their untreated disease state (and won't be until they get treated).
3. No help from health care, friends, employers, alcohol, drugs and family, and therefore depending on something outside that failed support system.

The contact with the individual concerning Christianity arose in an unusual manner. I was renting a home for $1600 CDN monthly and had an endless number of deficiencies in the house that were not addressed. I dealt directly with the owner and sales/lease agent with truthfully over 100 phone calls and emails. I threatened to go to the governmental agency mediating between landlords and tenants in the province and lo and behold I had a meeting with the president of the property agency handling the lease within days.

I had noticed that in emails his signature ended with Blessings. Keeping this in mind I went to the meeting and encountered, as I foresaw, a very defensive and rigid stance from the onset of our appointment. I also in truth began with a chip on the proverbial shoulder, but fifteen minutes into the conversation I suddenly interjected (don't know why, even now until the moment of writing this line!) with, "Are you a Christian?" He was befuddled for several moments and continued on with business. I pursued with the question and finally he answered in the affirmative.

We started to both relax and I revealed my sense of spirituality, and suddenly he poured out with struggles of his business, recent huge financial losses and the weekly struggle to make payroll. He said that he was feeling the Devil attacking at every glance. He spoke of a very small congregation that he and his second wife and two young children attended. It sounded very enticing and I truly felt the sincerity of his pouring out his personal story to a potential "difficult client".

We went on to discuss life and Christianity for over an hour, no business. I felt less urgent in my complaints.

He commented that he felt the power of the Holy Spirit in my coming that day and it was not as a client. I eventually attended his church a couple weeks later but in the intervening period he invited me to a lunchtime get together consisting of his Pastor, a spiritual advisor to him (happened to be his dentist as a child!) and myself (as a new spiritual presence in his life).

It was an honest and uplifting gathering of people who I had a heartfelt feeling, possessed a pure soul. Interestingly the dentist and I confessed to our major psychiatric pasts, him with severe depression (not bipolar) and me of course my complicated bipolar history.

I never felt treated differently subsequent to this "confession"...

The relationship with this individual and even his employees continued in earnest. An initial leasing agent who had contacted me with this firm, had "a husband dying of metastatic lung cancer". Although not practicing medicine at the time, I had had a hand in setting up the Palliative Care Unit in one of the major hospitals years before. A good colleague of mine still worked there and aided in getting direct admission for this man to die comfortably. Despite several attempts of my making arrangements and attempts at admitting him, the wife/employee never answered. She did however call me at 1:00 a.m. on several occasions, getting advice and then again never showing up for a palliative care bed, which had numerous dying individuals waiting for it. She was a "Christian".

I later found out from her boss – my "friend" – that she had defrauded his company of thousands of dollars, but stayed on the payroll for a time anyway! A reflection of how he managed his business. She was much later fired and disappeared "after the death" of her husband. The veracity of her entire story was put into question.

Well months went by, and I thought that my friend from 'communal faith and Christianity' would help me out with my house issues now six months in duration. Nothing.

I don't know if there was really a staffing issue, but my house had dangerous deficiencies and I had no choice but to go to the governmental tenant relations board after numerous unsuccessful attempts at contacting the owner, leasing agent and my church co-congregant. My suspicions were aroused when as a former soldier, I wanted to read a poem I had written one Sunday at the pulpit, to commemorate two soldiers slain by *mentally ill murderers who had sought mental health care within five years of the murders!*

I was told quote, through email, that the Pastor would have to politely decline "because he guarded the pulpit closely!" Should have been a red flag seen from kilometres away (we're metric here in Canada).

To summarize, a complaint to the Landlord and Tenant Board ensued. The hate, deceit, unprofessional and unChristian-like communications from my 'Christian' friend were unbelievable. In fact a lawyer with the Tribunal (offered to tenants) viewed his comments before the hearing and said, "I have never heard anything like this in my ten years with the Tribunal, and I would just get out of this house."

Several very unprofessional and libellous emails ensued from this God-fearing man, with some including out-and-out threats asking me to leave the property "if I was so unhappy". This was totally inappropriate in his position as a property manager. I launched a complaint with the regional Better Business Bureau.

The straw that broke the camel's back is that my Christian friend sent an email to an innocent third party alluding to "my health" as a reason for complaining and that I should get help (remember he knew of my past psychiatric history). This was without any justification in regards to me displaying any symptoms of any psychiatric recurrence. He also said in all truth "that *I* delayed the deficiency repairs because I was preoccupied by helping the 'dying' husband of the embezzler in his employ."

Legal counsel agrees that I am owed thousands without getting into the details. I will leave my lease early (the owner has agreed) and though I feel I should have my day in court, will not pursue things further because I have learned *"not to sweat the small stuff!"*

PEOPLE WITH MENTAL HEALTH DIAGNOSES MUST STAND UP FOR THEIR RIGHTS ...

... because likely society – including your health care providers – won't. Consult the Canadian Mental Health Association or the appropriate equivalent in your country for advice!

The 'Christian' friend has a certain diagnosis of a malignant psychiatric disorder called passive-aggressive personality.

Now I know that at this point you all are thinking or saying, "This Kumar guy thinks that everyone has a psychiatric diagnosis!"

The truth is that psychiatrists will tell you that 'like attracts like'. Throughout my medical career, I attracted patients who had not had positive experiences with their family doctors, sometimes those of a lifetime. There was simply no one else to take care of them. They often had concomitant psychiatric disorders; remember, 1:4 patients, treated or undiagnosed are statistically so. Once these were treated, our relationships went on swimmingly for the most part with the medical problems treated at the same time.[4]

The same holds true for the people that I have met in life. I feel that I have naturally, perhaps therapeutically, attracted people with mental health care issues. Besides, now as a broken record, Vegas dream-odds of meeting someone by chance with such a history is 20-25 per cent and higher with what we call in medical research, a pre-selection bias!

Therefore, a warning to those of us with mental health battles, proceed with caution in financial ventures and involvement with *organized* religion (to be contrasted greatly with personal faith and spirituality.)

Finally, what probably amounts to the biggest "kick in the teeth" of all my rejections regarding being an advocate for mental health care in the country, was when I approached the Executive Director of the Canadian Mental Health Association (CMHA) of Toronto and an Adjunct Professor at the University of Toronto. It was for a proposal for one of the largest non-corporate inspired events to promote mental health care destigmatization of the disease in the country.

His response was and I quote, "I have read through your book (quickly). Thank you for sharing your story with me. At this time we are not able to take on new advocacy or public education projects."

Not what one would like to hear from an executive for arguably what *should be one of the largest advocates* for mental health in the country!

The tally on the disinterest in mental health causes in *my* southwestern Ontario city is:

1. CEO of the regional hospital where I was a patient for fifteen months,
2. Former CEO of Ontario Hydro who is also the CEO of the regional economic and development corporation,

3. Area MPP (member of provincial legislature),
4. Dean and Student Union of local Law School
5. City Heritage and Arts Council
6. Nurses on the hospital ward that I spent fifteen months on and I have met two years after discharge.
7. Former doctor colleagues
8. 'Christian' brethren
9. 'Business' associates

Not a ringing endorsement for a part of the country that espouses itself as the banner-bearer for "the working people of Canada"!

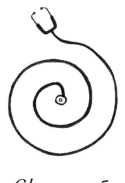

Chapter 5

THE BATTLE TO HAPPINESS PAUSES

In a temporal shift two to three years prior to the last part of Chapter 4...

A few months passed after discharge from the seniors' residence. I had moved into my rented condo and life was slowly returning to a semblance of normal. I was living independently but was still fighting all the battles I cited at the end of the last chapter.

A routine ultrasound of my neck, only ten months since my whole body radiation revealed several new lymph nodes on the left side of my neck that looked suspicious. A special thyroid scan showed no metastases to my lungs or bone. The biopsy was *positive for recurrent metastatic papillary thyroid carcinoma,* almost an unheard of recurrence after first treatment and never so soon (ten months) thereafter; normally there is a 95 per cent cure rate after the first treatment at 25 *years!)*

My faith and spirituality (two different things entirely) were being tested. By now I had little energy to fight yet another battle alone. As God would have it, a few months before the discovery of the cancer,

I was touring perspective doctor's offices (still at the very early stages of my medical licence marathon), when I was taken aback by a very energetic and attractive woman.[IX]

She within short order persuaded me to take a rescued mother and kitten to my condo, and made a special trip to deliver and "inspect her former charges' " new abode. The inspection lasted four hours with my homemade muffins and green tea!

To cut to the chase, we fell in love over the ensuing months. By the time of my cancer diagnosis and scheduled surgery, we had only known each other six months. The reality of the situation was that I could not live alone with my second cancer surgery in sixteen months (this time more extensive) and then the whole body radiation to follow. We came to the mutual conclusion that I should move in.

> "Beauty is not in the face; beauty is a light in the heart."
> —Kahlil Gibran

L. as I will call her, was fully aware of my past two years but very accepting. She rekindled in me a hearkening back to a sect of Hinduism that was a huge part of my now Canadianized culture, and reawakened Faith as a source for healing both emotionally and physically. However our budding romance was stressed by the shenanigans of the College, financial matters, my ex-wife's continuous harassment and L.'s own financial and occupational woes.

The relationship was doomed from the start, with the multitude of stressors never really allowing time for happiness, with endless bickering and character sniping. She was clearly distressed by the bipolar

---

IX Regardless of what political correctness dictates, 90 per cent of first attraction upon first meeting a member of the opposite sex is physical, as has been validated by study after study. This woman proved to be as attractive, if not more, inside!

disorder and my pointing out mental health issues in her family as well. Literature brought forth for her to understand my illness and her issues was angrily swept aside with clear evidence of denial and no desire to change the status quo. She was afraid of what would happen to her if I got sick and no amount of reassurance would do even with all the supports in place. Close examination of the nature of treated bipolar disease was never accepted.

In addition, I think that mental health issues of parental abandonment particularly by L.'s father, played a role in her ability to form male relationships. This came clearly to the fore in intensive couples' counseling but was never recognized, by L. admitted to, or addressed. In addition, *classic* co-dependency with both sons particularly the elder, were forever an issue swept under the rug with vehemence. Psychopathic tendencies and sexual identity questions almost acknowledged by the elder son himself were also a dark "secret" along with classic substance dependence issues in the younger son. The sum total of these mental health concerns was the wrench that destroyed the workings of a seemingly good match otherwise. There was a divergence in some things such as a conscious will to ignore world events on her part (ruined idyllic and exaggerated religious/faith dependence) and the non-pursuit of other academic interests that are important to me, which also played a part in the demise of the relationship.

Despite several heroic attempts at rekindling the initially strong bond, it dissolved under suboptimal circumstances. I cite the numerous issues described above as the "mysterious" causes for the problems. With the prevalence of mental health illness at 20 to 25 per cent in the general public, it's not surprising that the majority of romantic relationships end up in divorce/separation!

Despite all this, L. did help save my life and for that reason I will treasure the memories of our time together.

I survived the second cancer treatment but have developed other medical problems since that have hampered my health and for which I continue on disability Appendix 2.

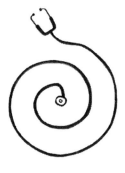

Chapter 6

BLISS!

It's now a little over three years since as I was discharged from hospital. Life is much better, though some of the consequences of improper mental health care, stigmatization, damage to my reputation and career are things that I struggle with daily.

I have fought back to recoup some ground in my career as can be read on my LinkedIn site in Appendix 4, my curriculum vitae, and obviously including this book. I have multiple medical research projects in progress, including my R.T. Medical Research/Advocacy Corporation[X] and a major charity initiative involving aboriginal Australian and First Nations' arts benefiting street people in our city, many of whom are psychiatric patients ignored by the system. I am also involved in co-writing a law for Ontario on patient rights and advocacy.

X   R.T. Kumar. Curriculum vitae under ABOUT THE AUTHOR. Accessed July 18, 2015. www.rtkumar.com

I have ongoing plans for a *huge* promotion of mental health patient rights in the planning stages, but this remains a surprise!

My struggle to regain my medical licence continues with the support of my psychiatrist, the PHP and a very supportive law firm.

I remain fanatically compliant with medication, on one occasion even driving four hours to an airport to start a very needed seven day vacation, getting to the airport and realizing I had not packed one of my medications, and turning around for home, sacrificing the money (and time away!) in favour of staying on my meds.

I would like to close my story with the following. If you suspect you have a mental health diagnosis *please seek help!* I have included in Appendix 5 several sites for helping and identifying mental health conditions.

If you are the relative, friend, loved one or even an acquaintance of someone who you strongly suspect has a mental health diagnosis, try and get them to a source of help. This is more often than not difficult due to denial. But when the person becomes a threat to themselves or someone else, the law intervenes and can be used to help, for example law enforcement bringing the patient to medical aid. As per my story and indicated otherwise throughout this book, the error of omission or inaction can be disastrous!

Although the tone of this book on the system's handling of mental health care is negative, the other side of the coin is that most workplaces now have EAPs as previously noted. These help with mental health care and substance dependence issues. Although the financial help during treatment and treatment itself varies, at least it's a foot in the door! Technically, according to federal legislation and human rights charters in our country, an individual cannot be discriminated against due to issues covered by EAPs. This however, in my medical experience, is still circumnavigated by firms where ignorance and stigma persists, and patients are sometimes 'let go' due to mental health disease but under totally another pretense.

Also remember that if you have substance dependence issues *seek help* for the 90 per cent chance you also have a mental health diagnosis!

Finally, I hope that if nothing else, I have illustrated that mental illness affects everyone, even us arrogant doctors who, like teenagers, feel we are invincible, or are too afraid for a myriad of reasons to seek help! (Doctor heal thyself!) The consequences of non-treatment and even inadequate or negligent treatment are almost always damaging on physical health, marital and familial relationships, occupation and most importantly *quality of life*! Now seemingly as a broken record, these consequences can be irreversible for the patient and their loved ones.

Please don't become a statistic.

I hope that this book saves even one life. If so, my reason for writing it will have been served. But I do have one last parting thought that I began with in the introduction.

THERE IS ALWAYS HOPE!

Even though this disease is one that deprives you of this very entity, it is the job of loved ones, "ideally" health care professionals, friends and others who care, to supplant this lifeline when you may think it will never exist again. In my case, you have heard how hope was something that was not present while I was acutely ill. But I can honestly say, that despite all that has happened to me since, I may lose hope for an evening.

But with the sunrise of the next day, whether it be divine intervention, stubborn determination or a will to live so strong now that it eclipses all else in my life, other than my never ending love for those who love me, THE HOPE IS BACK!

My hope – for me and all of us who live with mental health disease – will not waver!

I hope to continue in this vein with my next book, which will examine systematically where in society mental health care breaks down and perhaps how to fix it.

I end with a quote from the famous Lebanese poet Kahlil Gibran from his masterpiece "Defeat":

Defeat, my Defeat, my deathless courage,
You and I shall laugh together with the storm,
And together we shall dig graves for all that die in us,
And we shall stand in the sun with a will,
And we shall be dangerous...
—Kahlil Gibran

R.T. Kumar
January 17, 2015

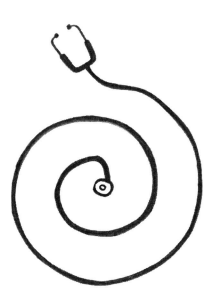

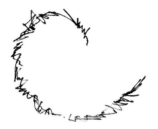

Endnotes

1. ECT still has a role in depression treatment today, though not as prevalent as in the 1960s and 70s when Mom was treated.

2. Nancy Andreasen. *The Creating Brain: The Neuroscience of Genius.* (New York: Dana Press, 2005), 197.

3. Bertram Stoffelmayr, Lois Benishek, Keith Humphrey, Julia Lee & Brian Mavis. "Substance Abuse Prognosis with an Additional Psychiatric Diagnosis: Understanding the Relationship." J Psychoactive Drugs. 1989 Apr-Jun; 21(2):145-52. www.ncbi.nlm.nih.gov/pubmed/2760755

4. Elie Elovic, Edgardo Baerga, Sara Cuccurullo (2004). "Traumatic brain injury." In Cuccurullo S.J. (Ed.) *Physical Medicine and Rehabilitation Board Review,* 54–55.

5. Sonja Puzic. "Catering to 'unattached' patients: Hospitalists care for those without doctors." *Windsor Star,* Sept. 11, 2009.

6. T. J. Lambert. "The medical care of people with psychosis." Med J Aust. 2009 Feb 16; 190(4):171-2.

7. S.A. Mayer. "Head injury." In: Rowland LP (Ed.) *Merritt's Neurology*. 11th Ed. (Baltimore: Lippincott Williams & Wilkins, 2005), chap 64.

8. A. P. John et al. "Prevalence of metabolic syndrome among Australians with severe mental illness. Med J Aust. 2009 Feb 16; 190(4):176-9.

9. William Styron, *Darkness Visible: A Memoir of Madness*. (New York: Vintage 1992), 6-7.

10. C. Harihar, P. Dasari, J.S. Srinivas. "Intramuscular ketamine in acute depression: A report on two cases." Indian J Psychiatry [serial online] 2013 [cited 2015 Jun 7]; 55:186-8. Available from: www.indianjpsychiatry.org/text.asp?2013/55/2/186/111461.

11. Annie Burns-Piper, Kevin Newman. "W5 uncovers 300 suicide deaths by patients in Canadian hospitals." CTV W5, Oct. 4, 2014. Accessed June 7, 2015. www.ctvnews.ca/w5/w5-uncovers-300-suicide-deaths-by-patients-in-canadian- hospitals-1.2038520.

12. Matt Schiavenza. "How an ISIS beheading might change Japan. *The Atlantic*, January 21, 2015.

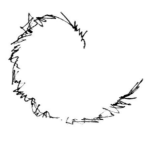

Appendix 1

FAMOUS PEOPLE WITH BIPOLAR DISORDER

The following is just a small sample of the many talented, creative and engaging people who have been diagnosed with Bipolar Disorder and gone on to lead successful lives.[XI]

>Russell Brand, actor
>Jim Carey, actor
>Robert Downey Jr., actor
>Carrie Fisher, author, actress, mental health activist
>Demi Lovato, singer and actress
>Sinéad O'Connor, singer/songwriter
>Jane Pauley, journalist
>Scott Stapp, musician

[XI] Everyday Health. "12 Famous People with Bipolar Disorder. Accessed July 18, 2015. www.everydayhealth.com/bipolar-disorder-pictures/famous-people-with-bipolar-disorder.aspx

Jean-Claude Van Damme, actor/writer/producer/director
Vincent van Gogh, artist
Charlie Sheen, actor
Virginia Woolf, author and essayist
Catherine Zeta-Jones, actress

OTHER ONLINE LIST RESOURCES:

en.wikipedia.org/wiki/List_of_people_with_bipolar_disorder

www.health.com/health/gallery/0,,20307117,00.html

www.mentalhealthadvocacyinc.org/role-models

www.mentalfloss.com/article/12500/11-historical-geniuses-and-their-possible-mental-disorders

www.adhdandbipolar.com/famous-people-with-bipolar-disorder.html

www.pinterest.com/bipolarbandit/famous-people-with-bipolar-disorder/

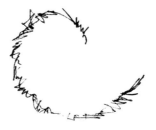

Appendix 2

MEDICAL HISTORY OF DR. R.T. KUMAR

This Appendix was written to show that patients with mental health diagnoses *sometimes* must deal with multiple complex medical problems, as well as coping with their psychiatric diagnosis. It has been documented by the World Psychiatric Association that people with severe mental illness have shorter lifespans compared to the general population.[XII] My physical conditions have included:

> Anemia (low blood)
> Blood clots both lungs
> Gallbladder (gangrenous)
> High cholesterol
> Impaired glucose tolerance (borderline diabetes)

[XII] Marc de Hurt et al. "Physical illness in patients with severe mental disorders. I. Prevalence, impact of medications and disparities in health care." *World Psychiatry*. 2011 Feb; 10(1): 52–77.

Low thyroid (after cancer treatment)
Low testosterone
Metastatic cancer of the thyroid twice (thyroid cancer
spread twice)
Mild decreased blood flow to heart
Mild kidney disease
Psoriasis (skin and joint disease)
Sleep apnea (stop breathing while sleeping)

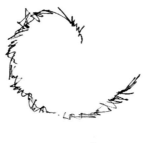

Appendix 3

INTERNET AND SOCIAL MEDIA MATERIAL ABOUT DR. R. T. KUMAR

SOURCES OF ACCURATE INFORMATION

Website clarifying libellous internet allegations
www.drtinnikumar.com

Official Website
www.rtkumar.com

Ontario Doctor Directory
www.ontariodoctordirectory.ca › … › Doctors in Chatham
Contact information and Free Ratings and Reviews for Dr. Rohit Tinni Kumar – Chatham, Ontario.

ServiceRating.ca [Medical Doctors]
mds.servicerating.ca/office/Rohit_Tinni_Kumar
Rohit Tinni Kumar is a medical practice in Ontario, Chatham. Search ServiceRating.ca for medical doctors. Rate them and share your experience with other...

mds.servicerating.ca/Dr/Rohit_Tinni_Kumar
Rohit Tinni Kumar is a medical doctor in Ontario, Chatham. Search ServiceRating.ca for medical doctors. Rate them and share your experience with other...

Dearborn, MI | Internal Medicine
www.doximity.com › States › Michigan › Dearborn
Dr. Rohit Kumar, MD is an internist in Dearborn, Michigan...

ZoomInfo
www.zoominfo.com/p/Rohit-Kumar/300475933
Dr. Rohit Tinni Kumar studied at Dalhousie University in Nova Scotia and interned at the Toronto East General and Orthopedic Hospital. He began his residency...

Chatham Daily News – *Kumar battles cancer*
www.chathamdailynews.ca/2010/08/27/kumar-battles-cancer
Aug 27, 2010 - Dr. Rohit Tinni Kumar wants his patients to know he didn't abandon them. In a brief interview with The Chatham Daily News Thursday...

SOURCES OF LIBELLOUS INFORMATION

Libelous material has been published on the Internet about Dr. Kumar with no examination of the full facts surrounding the claims. Several remain despite efforts to have them removed or corrected.

Chatham Daily News – The case of the missing doc
www.chathamdailynews.ca/2010/08/25/the-case-of-the-missing-doc
Aug 25, 2010 CHATHAM, ON – This is the Chatham office of Dr. Rohit Tinni Kumar on Grand Avenue. Kumar unexpectedly closed his family...

London Free Press – Doc's sex charge stayed for Year
www.lfpress.com/news/london/2010/09/17/15392081.html
Sep 17, 2010 – ... Rob MacDonald said in court Friday there are mental health issues involved in deciding to stay the charge against Dr. Rohit Tinni Kumar, 34.

Canoe – Virtual News Stand
virtual.canoe.ca/?type=291&publication=843151
Sept. 30, 2010 – COURT Charged stayed due to doctor's mental state ELLWOOD SHREVE ... in deciding to stay the charge against Dr. Rohit Tinni Kumar, 34.

Twitter – Blackburn News CK
www.twitter.com/blackburnck/status/24774422913
Sep 17, 2010 – court stays sexual assault charge against Dr. Tinni Kumar. 0 replies 0 retweets 0...

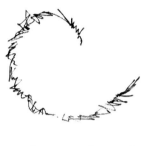

Appendix 4

SOCIAL MEDIA SITES BY OR ABOUT DR. KUMAR

General information:
www.rtkumar.com

LinkedIn:
Site can be found by searching LinkedIn under R.T. Kumar MD MSc Capt (ret'd)

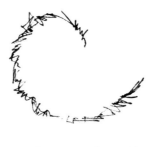

Appendix 5

HELPFUL SITES ON MENTAL HEALTH

Canadian Institute for Health Information
www.cihi.ca/CIHI-ext-portal/internet/
EN/Home/home/cihi000001

Canadian Mental Health Association
www.cmha.ca

Canadian Mental Health Association BC
www.cmha.bc.ca/get-informed/
mental-health-information/bipolar-disorder

Canadian Veterans Advocacy
www.canadianveteransadvocacy.com

Centre for Addiction and Mental Health
www.camh.ca/en/hospital/Pages/home.aspx

Courageous Companions (PTSD Dogs)
www.asist.ca/CourageousCompanions.html

Mental Health Canada
www.mentalhealthcanada.com/

Mental Health Commission of Canada
www.mentalhealthcommission.ca/

Mental Health Strategy for Canada:
A Youth Perspective (May 2015)
www.mentalhealthcommission.ca/English/document/72171/
mental-health-strategy-canada-youth-perspective

Mood Disorders Society of Canada
www.mooddisorderscanada.ca/

National Institute of Mental Health
www.nimh.nih.gov/health/topics/index.shtml

National Network for Mental Health
www.nnmh.ca

The Royal –
Women's Mental Health/
Operational Stress Injuries/PTSD
www.theroyal.ca/mental-health-centre/
mental-health-programs/areas-of-care/womens-mental-health/

True Patriot Love
truepatriotlove.com

Women's College Hospital –
Women's Mental Health Program

www.womenscollegehospital.ca/
programs-and-services/mental-health

Wounded Warriors Canada
woundedwarriors.ca/home/

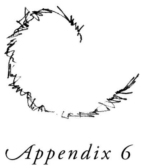

Appendix 6

CORPORATE ADVOCATES FOR MENTAL HEALTH CARE

Bell Canada – Let's Talk Community Fund
www.letstalk.bell.ca/en/our-initiatives/community-fund/how-to-apply/

Canada Post Community Foundation – Child and Youth Mental Health
www.canadapost.ca/cpo/mc/aboutus/cpfoundation/default.jsf

Great-West Life Centre for Mental Health in the Workplace
www.workplacestrategiesformentalhealth.com/

Lundbeck Canada Inc.
www.lundbeck.com/global/CSR/positions/mental-health

ScotiaBank – Centre for Addiction and Mental Health
www.camh.ca/en/hospital/about_camh/news-room/CAMH_in_the_headlines/stories/Pages/Scotiabank-gives-back-to-CAMH.aspx

Among many others!

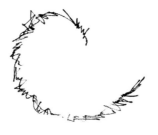

Sources

Nancy Andreasen (2005). In *The Creating Brain: The Neuroscience of Genius,* 97, 104.

Harry Hemingway and Michael Marmot. "Evidence based cardiology. Psychosocial factors in the aetiology and prognosis of coronary heart disease: systematic review of prospective cohort studies." *BMJ* 1999 318:146.

Elie Elovic, Edgardo Baerga and Sara Cuccurullo (2004). "Traumatic brain injury." In Cuccurullo S.J. (Ed.) *Physical Medicine and Rehabilitation Board Review,* 54–55.

Bertram Stoffelmayr, Lois Benishek, Keith Humphrey, Julia Lee and Brian Mavis. "Substance Abuse Prognosis with an Additional Psychiatric Diagnosis: Understanding the Relationship."
J Psychoactive Drugs 1989; Apr-Jun; 21(2):145-152.

Sonja Puzic. "Catering to 'unattached' patients: Hospitalists care for those without doctors." Windsor Star, September 11, 2009.

A.P. John, R. Koloth, M. Dragovic and L.C. Kim. "Prevalence of metabolic syndrome among Australians with severe mental illness." *Med J* Aust 2009; 190(4):176-9.

"Diabetes in Canada: Facts and figures from a public health perspective. Chapter 1- The burden of diabetes in Canada (2011)." Public Health Agency of Canada.

William Stryon (1992) In *Darkness Visible: A Memoir of Madness*. Quote from Goodreads Quotable Quotes.

Akira Kudoh, Yoko Takahira, Hiroshi Katagai and Tomoko Takazawa. "Small-dose Ketamine Improves the Postoperative State of Depressed Patients." *Anesth Analg* 2002; 95:114–8.

Annie Burns-Pieper and Kevin Newman. "W5 uncovers 300 suicide deaths by patients in Canadian hospitals." Accessed July 18, 2015. www.ctvnews.ca/w5/w5-uncovers-300-suicide-deaths-by-patients-in-canadian-hospitals-1.2038520

Debra Davis, Linda Luecken and Alex Zautra. "Are Reports of Child Abuse Related to the Experience of Chronic Pain in Adulthood? A Meta-analytic Review of the Literature." *Clinical Journal of Pain*: 2005; Sept-Oct; 21(5):398-405.

Peter Stoffer, M.P. Official Opposition Critic for Veterans Affairs, New Democratic Party. "Peter Soffer M.P. regarding Bill C-58 and the three proposed new benefits for veterans and their families." In *Canadian Veterans' Advocacy; one veteran one standard*. Accessed July 18, 2015. www.canadianveteransadvocacy.com/blog/?p=1297

"Mental health in the military: Ottawa to spend $200M over 6 years." CBC News online. Accessed July 18, 2015. www.cbc.ca/

news/politics/mental-health-in-the-military-ottawa-to-spend-200m-over-6-years-1.2846166.

"Auditor General 2014 report: Veterans' mental-health services criticized." CBC News online. Accessed July 18, 2015. www.cbc.ca/news/politics/auditor-general-2014-report-veterans-mental-health-services-criticized-1.2849021

"Suicide claims more soldiers than those killed by Afghan combat." The Star, September 16, 2014. Accessed July 18, 2015. www.thestar.com/news/canada/2014/09/16/suicide_claims_more_soldiers_than_those_killed_by_afghan_combat.html

"More Canadian than British soldiers took own lives in 2013." CBC News Accessed July 18, 2015. www.cbc.ca/news/world/more-canadian-than-british-soldiers-took-own-lives-in-2013-1.2604078

Igor Oyffe, Rena Kurs, Marc Gelpkopf, Yuval Melamed and Avi Bleich. "Revolving-door patients in a public psychiatric hospital in Israel: cross sectional study." *Croat Med J* 2009 December; 50(6): 575-582.

Stephen Kisely and Leslie Anne Campbell. "Does compulsory or supervised community treatment reduce 'revolving door' care? Legislation is inconsistent with recent evidence." *B J Psych* 2005; 191(5):304-05.

Fábio L Gastal, Sérgio B Andreoli, Maria Inês S Quintana, Maurício Almeida Gameiro, Sérgio O Leite and John McGrath. "Predicting the revolving door phenomenon among patients with schizophrenic, affective disorders and non-organic psychoses." *Rev. Saúde Pública* 2000; 34(3): 280-85.

David Dias Neto and Ana Catarina da Silva. "Characterization of readmissions at a Portuguese psychiatric hospital: An analysis over a 21 month period." *Eur J Psychiat* 2008; 22(2).

J. Rabinowitz, M. Mark, M. Popper, M. Slyuzberg and H. Munitz. "Predicting revolving-door patients in a 9-year national sample." *Soc Psychiatry Psychiatr Epidemiol* 1995; March 30(2):65-72.

P. Garrido and C.B. Saraiva. "P-601 - Understanding the revolving door syndrome." *J of the Europ Psych Assoc* 2012; Supplement 1, Page 1.

Marvin S. Swartz, Jeffrey W. Swanson, H. Ryan Wagner, Barbara J. Burns, Virginia A. Hiday and Randy Borum. "Can Involuntary Outpatient Commitment Reduce Hospital Recidivism? Findings from a Randomized Trial with Severely Mentally Ill Individuals." *Amer J of Psych.* 1999; 156(12):1968-1975.

Andrea E Williamson, Paul CD Johnson, Kenneth Mullen and Philip Wilson. "The disappearance of the 'revolving door' patient in Scottish general practice: successful policies." *BMC Family Practice* 2012, 13:95

Wayne Weiten (2007). *"Mental Illness, the Revolving Door."* In *Psychology: Themes and Variations: Themes And Variations, 623-24.*

"Military's mental health system 'abandoned' CFB Shilo soldier." CBC NewsAccessed July 18, 2015. www.cbc.ca/news/canada/manitoba/military-s-mental-health-system-abandoned-cfb-shilo-soldier-1.2797515.

"Veterans' mental health: more funding needed, says PTSD expert." CBC News Accessed July 18, 2015. www.cbc.ca/news/canada/british-columbia/

veterans-mental-health-more-funding-needed-says-ptsd-expert-1.2849621

"Calgary skyscraper attack plotter contacted Veterans Affairs for help." CBC News. Accessed July 18, 2015. www.cbc.ca/news/canada/calgary/calgary-skyscraper-attack-plotter-contacted-veterans-affairs-for-help-1.2827039

"Ron Francis's lawyer makes plea for PTSD help after Mountie's suicide." CBC News. Accessed July 18, 2015. www.cbc.ca/news/canada/new-brunswick/ron-francis-s-lawyer-makes-plea-for-ptsd-help-after-mountie-s-suicide-1.2789975

Kirsten Patrick. "Depression deserves better treatment." *CMAJ* 2014;186:1043.

Matt Schiavenza. "How an ISIS beheading may change Japan." *The Atlantic*. Accessed July 18, 2015. www.theatlantic.com/international/archive/2015/01/how-an-isis-beheading-might-change-japan/384806/

Lightning Source UK Ltd.
Milton Keynes UK
UKOW02f0352030616

275483UK00001B/108/P